Dental and Otolaryngology Word Book

Helen E. Littrell, CMT

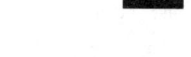

Springhouse
Word Book Series

Springhouse Corporation
Springhouse, Pennsylvania

© Copyright 1992 by
Springhouse Corporation
1111 Bethlehem Pike
Springhouse, Pennsylvania 19477

All rights reserved. No part of this book may be reproduced, stored in a retrieval system or transmitted in any form or by any means, electronic, mechanical, photocopying, recording or otherwise, without written permission from the publisher, except for brief quotations embodied in critical articles and reviews.

Printed in the United States of America

Library of Congress Catalog Card Number: 91-5130

ISBN: 0-87434-476-X

SWB 14-010192

Dedication

To my boys: Bryan, Kenneth, Bo, and Mitt

Success becomes a reality when you consider
each stumbling block as a stepping stone.

How to use this book

All entries in this book are listed alphabetically. When a term may be modified in some way by a variety of other terms, the sub-entries are indented and punctuated as follows:
   adenoma (main entry)
      chief cell a. (main entry comes after sub-entry)
      gelatinosum, a. (main entry comes before sub-entry)

We've also provided extensive cross-referencing to help you locate certain terms more easily. You'll find this especially valuable when abbreviations may be used interchangeably with the full entry: for example, TMJ (temporomandibular joint) is also listed as temporomandibular joint (TMJ).

As an added value, plural forms of words which change due to Latin origin are shown in parentheses following the root word, for example: foramen (pl. foramina). Foramina (pl. of foramen) is also listed alphabetically.

Also included in this book are many coined words and phrases, as well as medical slang. Because some of these terms are unconventional, you are unlikely to find them presented in other reference books. This is why they are part of this book; medical professionals must have a comprehensive reference source for the unique terms that are becoming more and more a part of their daily lives.

Acknowledgments

My deepest appreciation goes to all of those who assisted me with this book. I am very grateful to each of you for your understanding and support. Special thanks goes to Joel P. Slaughter, D.M.D. and Evelyn Rowland for their help.

Additionally, it's a distinct privilege to work with the staff at Springhouse Corporation, especially Jean Robinson and Wendy Clarke, who have been so helpful throughout the publication process.

I also wish to mention a longtime friend, G.P., who has demonstrated over and over that true friendship is not limited by distance. Thank you for being there whenever I needed you.

Finally, I must acknowledge my readers, for without you, there would have been no reason for me to write this book and the others in the series. Each one of you is very important to me.

Helen E. Littrell, CMT

Aarskog syndrome
Aarskog-Scott syndrome
Aase syndrome
aasmus
AB (axiobuccal)
Abadie sign
Abbe
    flap, A.
    operation, A.
Abbe-Estlander flap
Abbott esophagogastrectomy
ABC (airway-breathing-circulation or axiobuccocervical)
abdominal
    asthma, a.
    esophagus, a.
abducens
    labiorum, a.
    oculi, a.
abducent
Abelson
    adenotome, A.
    cricothyrotomy cannula, A.
    cricothyrotomy trocar, A.
aberrant
    goiter, a.
ABG (axiobuccogingival)
ABL (axiobuccolingual)
ablate
ablation
ablative laser therapy
ABLB (alternate binaural loudness balance)
    test, A.
abocclusion
aborad
aboral
ABR (auditory brain stem evoked response)
Abraham
    laryngeal cannula, A.
    tonsil knife, A.
Abrami disease

abrasion
abrasive
    disk, a.
abrasor
abscess
    alveolar a.
    apical a.
    Bezold a.
    blind a.
    circumtonsillar a.
    dental a.
    dentoalveolar a.
    dural a.
    extradural a.
    gingival a.
    intramastoid a.
    lacrimal a.
    masticator a.
    mastoid a.
    orbital a.
    otic cerebral a.
    palatal a.
    parapharyngeal a.
    parietal a.
    parotid a.
    periapical a.
    pericemental a.
    pericoronal a.
    peridental a.
    periodontal a.
    peritonsillar a.
    phoenix a.
    prelacrimal a.
    pulp a.
    pulpal a.
    retropharyngeal a.
    retrotonsillar a.
    root a.
    subdural a.
    subperiosteal a.
    Thornwaldt a.
    tonsillar a.
    tooth a.

abscess *(continued)*
    Tornwaldt a.
    tympanocervical a.
    tympanomastoid a.
    von Bezold a.
abscission
abutment
    auxiliary a.
    implant a.
    intermediate a.
    isolated a.
    multiple a.
    primary a.
    secondary a.
    terminal a.
abutment locator
abutment post
abutment splint
abutment tooth
AC (air conduction or axiocervical)
ACA (anticentromere antibody)
acalcerosis
acalcicosis
acanthiomeatal line
acanthion
accessional tooth
accessory
    cartilage of nose, a.
    maxillary hiatus, a.
    palatine canals, a.
    parotid gland, a.
    teeth, a.
    thyroid gland, a.
    tonsil, a.
accipiter
ACCO orthodontic appliance
accretion lines
achalasia
acheilia
acheilous
acid etching
acidogenic theory
acidosis
acidotic
acinar cell adenocarcinoma
Acinetobacter

Acinetobacter *(continued)*
    lwoffi, A.
Ackerman bar
ACMI
    bronchoscope, A.
    nasopharyngoscope, A.
acne
    keloid, a.
acneiform
Acorn nebulizer
acouesthesia
acoumeter
acoumetry
acouometer
acouophone
acouophonia
acousma
acoustic
    aphasia, a.
    apparatus, a.
    area, a.
    center, a.
    crest, a.
    duct, a.
    hair cells, a.
    immitance, a.
    labyrinth, a.
    meatal flap, a.
    meatus, a.
    nerve, a.
    neurilemoma, a.
    neurinoma, a.
    neuroma, a.
    neurotomy, a.
    organ, a.
    reflex, a.
    trauma deafness, a.
    tumor, a.
    window, a.
acousticofacial
    crest, a.
    ganglion, a.
acousticon
acousticophobia
acoustics
acquired cuticle

acrodynia
acrofacial dysostosis
acromegaly
acromicria
Acrotorque hand engine
acrylic
   resin, a.
   resin base, a.
   splint, a.
Actinomyces
   israelii, A.
actinomycosis
actinomycotin
activated resin
activator
   bow a.
   functional a.
   monoblock a.
acuity
   auditory a.
acupuncture/transcutaneous nerve stimulation (ACUTENS)
acusection
acusticus
acute
   bronchitis, a.
   catarrhal laryngitis, a.
   catarrhal tonsillitis, a.
   ear, a.
   laryngotracheobronchitis, a.
   necrotizing ulcerative gingivitis, a. (ANUG)
   pharyngitis, a.
ACUTENS (acupuncture/transcutaneous nerve stimulation)
AD (axiodistal or right ear)
Adam's apple
adamantine
adamantinocarcinoma
adamantinoma
adamantoblast
adamantoblastoma
adamantoma
adamanto-odontoma
adamas

adamas *(continued)*
   dentis, a.
Adams
   clasp, A.
   crushing procedure, A.
   otoplasty, A.
adaptation
adaxial
ADC (axiodistocervical)
Addis count
Addix needle and tier
adenalgia
adenectomy
adenectopia
adenia
adeniform
adenitis
   cervical a.
adenization
adenoameloblastoma
adenoangiosarcoma
adenoblast
adenocele
adenocellulitis
adenochondroma
adenochondrosarcoma
adenocyst
adenocystoma
adenocyte
adenodynia
adenoepithelioma
adenofibroma
   edematodes, a.
adenofibrosis
adenogenous
adenography
adenohypophysectomy
adenohypophysial
adenohypophysis
adenoid
   band, a.
   cystic carcinoma, a.
   face, a.
   facies, a.
   fossa, a.
   hypertrophy, a.

4 adenoid

adenoid *(continued)*
    pad, a.
    punch, a.
    tissue, a.
    tonsil, a.
adenoidectomy
adenoidism
adenoiditis
adenoids
adenolipoma
adenolipomatosis
adenolymphitis
adenolymphocele
adenolymphoma
adenoma
    adamantinum, a.
    alveolare, a.
    bronchial a's
    chief cell a.
    follicular a.
    gelatinosum, a.
    oxyphil a.
    pleomorphic a.
    serous cell a.
adenomalacia
adenomatoid
adenomatome
adenomatosis
    oris, a.
adenomatous
    goiter, a.
adenomegaly
adenoncus
adenoneural
adenopathy
adenopharyngitis
adenophlegmon
adenosclerosis
adenosis
adenotome
adenotomy
adenotonsillectomy
adenous
adenoviral
adenovirus
ADG (axiodistogingival)

adherent tongue
adhesive
    dental a.
    denture a.
adhesive otitis media
ADI (axiodistoincisal)
aditus
    ad antrum, a.
    ad antrum mastoideum, a.
    ad antrum tympanicum, a.
    glottidis inferior, a.
    glottidis superior, a.
    laryngis, a.
Adler attic ear punch
admaxillary gland
adnexa
    dental a.
    mastoidea, a.
ADO (axiodisto-occlusal)
adoral
Adson forceps
adult
    laryngoscope, a.
    respiratory distress syndrome, a. (ARDS)
    reverse-bevel laryngoscope, a.
advancement
    mandibular a.
advancement flap
adventitia
adventitious
    breath sounds, a.
    dentin, a.
AE (aryepiglottic)
    fold, A.
Aeby plane
AER (auditory evoked response)
aeration
aeroallergen
AeroChamber
aerodontalgia
aerodontia
aerodontics
aeroembolism
aero-odontalgia
aero-odontodynia

aero-otitis
aeropathy
aerophagia
aerosialophagy
aerosinusitis
aerosol
   bronchography, a.
   inhaler, a.
   spray, a.
aerosolization
aerosolized mist
aerotitis
aerotympanal conduction
Aesculap saw
Afrin nasal spray
afterhearing
aftertaste
AG (axiogingival)
agenesis
ageusic aphasia
agger (pl. aggeres)
   nasi, a.
   nasi cells, a.
   perpendicularis, a.
aggeres (pl. of agger)
aglossia
   -adactyly syndrome, a.
aglossostomia
aglutition
agnathia
agnathous
agnathus
agomphiasis
agomphious
agomphosis
agranulocytosis
Agrikola lacrimal sac retractor
AI (axioincisal)
air
   -bone gap, a.
   cell, a.
   conduction, a.
   -fluid level, a.
   hunger, a.
   swallowing, a.
   tube, a.

airborne
   allergen, a.
Air-Lon
   laryngectomy tube, A.
   tracheal tube, A
   tracheal tube brush, A.
airway
   esophageal obturator a.
   nasopharyngeal a.
   oropharyngeal a.
airway-breathing-circulation (ABC)
akinetic mutism
AL (axiolingual)
ala (pl. alae)
   auris, a.
   cristae galli, a.
   ethmoid, a. of
   major ossis sphenoidalis, a.
   minor ossis sphenoidalis, a.
   nasi, a.
   vomeris, a.
ALA (axiolabial)
alacrima
alae (pl. of ala)
ALAG (axiolabiogingival)
ALAL (axiolabiolingual)
alalia
alar
   cartilage, a.
   -columella implant, a.
   flaring, a.
   rim, a.
   scapula, a.
alarplasty
alaryngeal
   speech, a.
alate
ALB (alternate loudness balance)
Albers-Schonberg disease
Albert slotted bronchoscope
Albert-Andrews laryngoscope
Albinus muscle
Albright syndrome
albuminoid sputum
ALC (axiolinguocervical)
Alexander

Alexander *(continued)*
   chisel, A.
   deafness, A.
   gouge, A.
   mastoid chisel, A.
   otoplasty, A.
   otoplasty knife, A.
   tonsil needle, A.
Alezzandrini syndrome
ALG (axiolinguogingival)
alignment
   curve, a.
alimentary
   bolus, a.
   canal, a.
   tract, a.
alimentation
alinasal
alinement
aliquot
alisphenoid
   area, a.
   canal, a.
Alkolol nasal cleansing
allergen
allergenic
allergic
   asthma, a.
   cold, a.
   coryza, a.
   response, a.
   rhinitis, a.
   salute, a.
   shiner, a.
allergization
allergize
allergoid
allergosis
allergy
allicin
alligator forceps
Allis clamp
Allis-Coakley
   tonsil forceps, A.
   tonsil-seizing forceps, A.
Allis-Ochsner tonsil-forceps

Allison gastroesophageal reflux operation
Allium
all-metal ear syringe
allograft
alloplastic tooth
allotransplantation
allotriodontia
allotriogeustia
allotriophagy
allotriosmia
allylguaiacol
Almeida disease
Almoor extrapetrosal drainage procedure
Allport
   eustachian bur, A.
   gauze packer, A.
   incus hook, A.
   mastoid searcher, A.
   mastoid sound, A.
   syndrome, A.
   technique, A.
Allport-Babcock mastoid searcher
ALO (axiolinguo-occlusal)
Alstrom disease
Alsus-Knapp eyelid repair
Altenaria
alternate
   binaural loudness balance, a. (ABLB)
alternobaric vertigo
   loudness balance, a. (ALB)
alveobronchiolitis
alveobronchitis
Alveograf
alveolabial
alveolalgia
alveolar
   angle, a.
   arch, a.
   asthma, a.
   bone, a.
   canal, a.
   cavity, a.
   cleft, a.
   crest, a.
   gingiva, a.
   periosteum, a.

alveolar *(continued)*
    process of maxilla, a.
    ridge, a.
    segment, a.
alveolate
alveolectomy
alveoli (pl. of alveolus)
    dentales, a.
alveolitis
    sicca dolorosa, a.
alveoloclasia
alveolodental
    osteoperiostitis, a.
    periodontium, a.
alveololabial
alveololabialis
alveololingual
alveolomerotomy
alveolonasal
alveolopalatal
alveoloplasty
alveolotomy
alveolus (pl. alveoli)
    dental a.
    dentalis, a.
Alvis technique
AM (axiomesial)
ama
amalgam
    dental a.
    retrograde a.
amalgam carver
amalgam die
amalgam filling
amalgam plugger
amalgam tattoo
amalgamable
amalgamate
amalgamation
amalgamator
amaurotic nystagmus
ambient
    noise, a.
ambiguospinothalamic paralysis
ambiguous nucleus
amblyacousia

amblygeustia
amblyopic nystagmus
ambos
Ambu bag
AMC (axiomesiocervical)
AMD (axiomesiodistal)
AME PinSite Shields
amelification
ameloblast
ameloblastoma
amelodentinal
amelogenesis
    imperfecta, a.
amelogenic
amelogenin
American Sign Language (Ameslan)
Ameslan (American Sign Language)
amethocaine lozenge
AMG (axiomesiogingival)
AMI (axiomesioincisal)
Ammon
    blepharoplasty, A.
    canthoplasty, A.
    dacryocystotomy, A.
    triangle method, A.
amnemonic aphasia
amnesic aphasia
amnestic aphasia
AMO (axiomesio-occlusal)
amphicrania
amphidiarthrosis
amphoric voice
amphoriloquy
amphorophony
amplification
amplifier
ampulla (pl. ampullae)
ampullae (pl. of ampulla)
amusia
amygdala
    accessoria, a.
amygdaline
amygdaloid
amyloid tongue
anachoretic pulpitis
anacusia

anacusis
anakhre
anakusis
anallergic
anaphylactic crisis
anaphylactoid crisis
anastomosis
    Galen a.
    Jacobson a.
anchor
    endostial implant a.
anchor band
anchor splint
anchorage
    cervical a.
    compound a.
    extramaxillary a.
    extraoral a.
    intermaxillary a.
    intraoral a.
    maxillomandibular a.
    multiple a.
    occipital a.
    reciprocal a.
    reinforced a.
    simple a.
    stationary a.
ancipital
Andersch
    ganglion, A.
    nerve, A.
Anderson
    antrum punch, A.
    columella prosthesis, A.
    nasal strut, A.
    procedure, A.
Andresen appliance
Andrews
    applicator, A.
    bridge bar, A.
    ear applicator, A.
    gouge, A.
    laryngoscope, A.
    mastoid gouge, A.
    nasal applicator, A.
    tongue depressor, A.

Andrews *(continued)*
    tonsil forceps, A.
    tonsil-seizing forceps, A.
    tracheal retractor, A.
Andrews-Hartmann
    ear rongeur, A.
    forceps, A.
Andy Gump facies
anechoic room
Anel
    dilation of lacrimal duct, A.
    probe, A.
Angelchik anti-reflux prosthesis
Angelucci technique
aneurysmal
    bone cyst, a.
    cough, a.
angina
    catarrhalis, a.
    crouposa, a.
    epiglottidea, a.
    exudative a.
    follicularis, a.
    gangrenosa, a.
    hippocratic a.
    lacunar a.
    laryngea, a.
    Ludwig a.
    malignant a.
    membranacea, a.
    nosocomii, a.
    phlegmonosa, a.
    Plaut a.
    Plaut-Vincent a.
    pseudomembranous a.
    scarlatinosa, a.
    simplex, a.
    tonsillaris, a.
    trachealis, a.
    ulcerosa, a.
    Vincent a.
anginal
anginophobia
angiocheiloscope
angioedema
angiofibroma

angiofibroma *(continued)*
    juvenile a.
    nasopharyngeal a.
angioma
angioneurotic edema
angiopathic vertigo
angle
    alveolar a.
    auriculo-occipital a.
    axial a.
    axial line a.
    Bennett a.
    Broca a.
    buccal a's
    cavity a's
    cavosurface a.
    cephalic a.
    cephalometric a.
    chi a.
    convexity, a. of
    craniofacial a.
    cusp a.
    cusp plane a.
    Daubenton a.
    distal a's
    ethmocranial a.
    ethmoid a.
    facial a.
    gonial a.
    horizontal a.
    incisal a.
    incisal guide a.
    incisal mandibular plane a.
    Jacquart a.
    jaw, a. of
    labial a's
    line a.
    lingual a's
    mandible, a. of
    mandibular a.
    mastoid a. of parietal bone
    maxillary a.
    mesial a's
    metafacial a.
    mouth, a. of
    Mulder, a. of

angle *(continued)*
    nu a.
    occipital a.
    olfactive a.
    olfactory a.
    ophryospinal a.
    orifacial a.
    parietal a.
    Pirogoff a.
    point a.
    Quatrefage a.
    Ranke a.
    Serres a.
    sigma a.
    sphenoid a.
    squint a.
    tooth a's
    Topinard a.
    venous a.
    Virchow, a. of
    Vogt a.
    Weisbach a.
angle board
Angle
    classification, A.
    splint, A.
angophrasia
angular
    artery, a.
    cheilitis, a.
    cheilosis, a.
    elevator, a.
angulus
    mandibulae, a.
    mastoideus ossis parietalis, a.
    oris, a.
anhydrotic ectodermal dysplasia
anise oil
anisodont
ankyloblepharon
ankylocheilia
ankyloglossia
    complete a.
    partial a.
    superior, a.
ankylosed

ankylosed *(continued)*
    tooth, a.
ankylosis
    cricoarytenoid joint a.
    dental a.
    stapedial a.
ankylotia
ankylotic
ankylotome
ankylotomy
anlage
annealing
    lamp, a.
annular
    ligament, a.
annuli (pl. of annulus)
annulus (pl. annuli)
    tracheae, a.
    tympanic a.
    tympanicus, a.
    Vieussen a.
anodmia
anodontia
    partial a.
    true a.
    vera, a.
anodontism
anomic aphasia
anorexia
    nervosa, a.
anosmatic
anosmia
    gustatoria, a.
    preferential a.
    respiratoria, a.
anosmic
    aphasia, a.
anosmous
anosphrasia
anotia
anotus
ansa (pl. ansae)
    cervicalis, a.
    hypoglossi, a.
ansae (pl. of ansa)
ansiform

Antabuse
antagonist
antasthmatic
antegonial
    angle, a.
    notch, a.
anterior
    facial height, a.
    maxillary bowing sign, a.
    pillar, a.
    triangle, a.
anteroclusion
anthelix
Anthony
    mastoid suction tube, A.
    pillar retractor, A.
Anthony-Fisher antrum balloon
antiamebic
antibiotic
anticentromere antibody (ACA)
anticholinergic
antidinic
antifungal
antigen
antigenic
antihistamine
antihistaminic
antimicrobial
anti-Monson curve
antimycotic
antiniad
antinial
antinion
antiodontalgic
antipyogenic
antireflux prosthesis
antisialagogue
antisialic
antispasmodic
antitension lines (ATL)
antitragus
antitrismus
antitussive
    centrally-acting a.
antiviral
antra (pl. of antrum)

antral
   sinus cannula, a.
   wash tube, a.
   window, a.
antrectomy
antritis
antroatticotomy
antro-aural fistula
antrobuccal
antrocele
antrochoanal polyp
antrodynia
antronalgia
antronasal
antrophore
antrosaucerization
antroscope
antroscopy
antrostomy
   punch, a.
antrotome
antrotomy
antrotympanic
antrotympanitis
antrum (pl. antra)
   attic-aditus a.
   auris, a.
   cardiac a.
   cardiacum, a.
   ethmoid a.
   ethmoidale, a.
   frontal a.
   Highmore, a. of
   highmori, a.
   mastoid a.
   mastoideum, a.
   maxillare, a.
   maxillary a.
   tympanic a.
   tympanicum, a.
antrum balloon
antrum bur
antrum curette
antrum-exploring needle
antrum gouge
antrum-irrigating tube

antrum punch
antrum rasp
antrum wash tube
antrum window procedure
ANUG (acute necrotizing ulcerative gingivitis)
anulus
   tympanicus, a.
anvil
AO (axio-occlusal)
aosmic
AP (axiopulpal)
apatite
   crystal, a.
Apert syndrome
apertognathia
apertura (aperturae)
   chordae tympani, a.
   externa aqueductus vestibuli, a.
   sinus frontalis, a.
   sinus sphenoidalis, a.
   tympanica canaliculi, a.
aperturae
aperture
   anterior nasal a.
   frontal sinus, a. of
   glottis, a. of
   larynx, a. of
   sphenoid sinus, a.
   tympanic a. of canaliculus of chorda tympani
apex (pl. apices)
   arytenoid cartilage, a. of
   auriculae, a.
   cartilaginis arytenoideae, a.
   cuspidis, a.
   linguae, a.
   nasi, a.
   radicis dentis, a.
aphagia
   algera, a.
aphagic
aphagopraxia
aphasia
   acoustic a.
   ageusic a.

aphasia *(continued)*
   amnemonic a.
   amnesic a.
   amnestic a.
   anomic a.
   anosmic a.
   associative a.
   ataxic a.
   auditory a.
   Broca a.
   central a.
   combined a.
   commissural a.
   complete a.
   conduction a.
   cortical a.
   expressive a.
   expressive-receptive a.
   fluent a.
   frontocortical a.
   frontolenticular a.
   functional a.
   gibberish a.
   global a.
   graphomotor a.
   Grashey a.
   impressive a.
   intellectual a.
   jargon a.
   Kussmaul a.
   lenticular a.
   lethica, a.
   Lichtheim a.
   mixed a.
   motor a.
   nominal a.
   nonfluent a.
   optic a.
   parieto-occipital a.
   pathematic a.
   pictorial a.
   psychosensory a.
   receptive a.
   semantic a.
   sensory a.
   subcortical a.

aphasia *(continued)*
   syntactical a.
   tactile a.
   temporoparietal a.
   total a.
   transcortical a.
   traumatic a.
   true a.
   verbal a.
   visual a.
   Wernicke a.
aphasic
aphasiologist
aphasiology
aphemesthesia
aphemia
aphonia
   clericorum, a.
   hysterical a.
   paralytica, a.
   paranoica, a.
   spastic a.
aphonic
aphonogelia
aphrasia
aphtha (pl. aphthae)
aphthae (pl. of aphtha)
   Bednar a.
   cachectic a.
aphthobulbar stomatitis
aphthoid
aphthongia
aphthosis
aphthous
   stomatitis, a.
   ulceration, a.
apical
   abscess, a.
   base, a.
   curettage, a.
   elevator, a.
   periodontal cyst, a.
   pick, a.
apicoectomize
apicectomy
apices (pl. of apex)

apicitis
apicoectomy
apicostomy
apicotomy
apnea
    deglutition a.
    initial a.
    late a.
    neonatorum, a.
    posthyperventilation a.
    sleep a.
    traumatic a.
apnea alarm mattress
apnea monitor
apneic
    oxygenation, a.
    spell, a.
aponeurosis
    epicranial a.
    lingual a.
    palatine a.
    pharyngeal a.
aponeurositis
aponeurotic
aponeurotome
aponeurotomy
apophlegmatic
apophysary
apophyseal
apophyseopathy
apophyses (pl. of apophysis)
apophysis (pl. apophyses)
    Ingrassias, a. of
    Rau, a. of
apoplectic vertigo
apoplectiform deafness
aposia
apositia
aposthematous cheilitis
apparatus
    acoustic a.
    auditory a.
    digestive a.
    lacrimal a.
    masticatory a.
    respiratory a.

apparatus *(continued)*
    sound-conducting a.
    sound-perceiving a.
    vocal a.
apple-packer's epistaxis
apple-picker's disease
appliance
    ACCO orthodontic a.
    Andresen a.
    Begg a.
    Bimler a.
    craniofacial a.
    Crozat a.
    Denholz a.
    edgewise a.
    expansion plate a.
    extraoral a.
    fixed a.
    Frankel a.
    habit-breaking a.
    Hawley a.
    Jackson a.
    Johnson twin wire a.
    jumping-the-bite a.
    Kesling a.
    Kingsley a.
    labiolingual a.
    monoblock a.
    orthodontic a.
    permanent a.
    prosthetic a.
    removable a.
    ribbon arch a.
    Schwarz a.
    split plate a.
    twin wire a.
    universal a.
    Walker a.
applicator
apraxia
aprismatic enamel
apsithyria
aptyalia
apytalism
Aquaplast splint
aqueduct

aqueduct *(continued)*
    cochlea, a. of
    cochlear a.
    Cotunnius, a. of
    fallopian a.
    Fallopius, a. of
    vestibular a.
    vestibule, a. of
aqueductus
    cochleae, a.
    endolymphaticus, a.
    Fallopii, a.
    vestibuli, a.
aqueous zephiran
arachidic bronchitis
arachnorhinitis
arbor bronchialis
Arbuckle
    antral knife, A.
    antral saw, A.
    sinus probe, A.
Arcelin view
arch
    alveolar a.
    auricular a.
    branchial a's
    carotid a.
    Corti, a's of
    dental a.
    glossopalatine a.
    hyoid a.
    jugular a.
    lingual a.
    malar a.
    mandibular a.
    maxillary a.
    nasal a.
    oral a.
    palatal a.
    palatine a.
    palatoglossal a.
    palatomaxillary a.
    palatopharyngeal a.
    palpebral a.
    passive lingual a.
    pharyngeal a's

arch *(continued)*
    pharyngoepiglottic a.
    pharyngopalatine a.
    postaural a's
    residual dental a.
    ribbon a.
    right aortic a.
    stationary lingual a.
    supraorbital a.
    thyrohyoid a.
    zygomatic a.
arch bars
arch form
arch width
arch wire
archaeocerebellum
archaeocortex
archeocerebellum
archeocortex
archipallium
arcuate
    crest, a.
    eminence, a.
arcus
    alveolaris mandibulae, a.
    alveolaris maxillae, a.
    dentalis, a.
    glossopalatinus, a.
    lipoides myringis, a.
    palatini, a.
    palatoglossus, a.
    palatopharyngeus, a.
    pharyngopalatinus, a.
    zygomaticus, a.
ARDS (adult respiratory distress syndrome)
area
    acoustic a.
    acustica, a.
    alisphenoid a.
    auditory a.
    basal seat a.
    Broca motor speech a.
    Broca parolfactory a.
    cochleae, a.
    cochlear a.

area *(continued)*
    cribrosa media, a.
    denture-bearing a.
    denture foundation a.
    denture-supporting a.
    facial nerve, a. of
    hypoglossal a.
    hypoglossi, a.
    impression a.
    Kiesselbach a.
    Laimer-Haeckerman a.
    Little a.
    mesobranchial a.
    nervi facialis, a.
    olfactory a.
    post dam a.
    posterior palatal seal a.
    pterygoidea, a.
    relief a.
    rest a.
    rugae a.
    saddle a.
    stress-bearing a.
    supporting a.
    vestibular a.
    vestibularis inferior, a.
    vestibularis superior, a.
    vocal a.
    Wernicke a.
Arenberg-Denver inner ear valve
areola
areolar
    gingiva, a.
    tissue, a.
argon laser
argyria
    nasalis, a.
arhinencephalia
arhinia
Armdorfer esophageal motility probe
Armour endotracheal tube
Armstrong-Schuknecht stapes prosthesis
Arnold
    auricular ganglion, A.
    canal, A.
    ligament, A.

Arnold *(continued)*
    nerve, A.
    nerve reflex cough syndrome, A.
Aronson-Fletcher antrum cannula
arrested caries
arrow clasp
Arrow-Howes multilumen catheter
arrow-point tracing
arrowhead clasp
Arslan fenestration procedure
arteria
    stapedia, a.
arteritis
arthritis
    cricoarytenoid a.
    rheumatoid a.
arthrometric cephalostat
arthroplasty
    gap a.
    interposition a.
    intracapsular temporomandibular joint a.
arthroscopic
arthroscopy
articular
    lip, a.
    surface, a.
articulare
articulate
articulating paper
articulatio (pl. articulationes)
articulation
    articulator a.
    balanced a.
    cricoarytenoid a.
    cricothyroid a.
    incudomalleolar a.
    incudostapedial a.
    mandibular a.
    maxillary a.
    temporomandibular a.
    temporomaxillary a.
articulationes (pl. of articulatio)
articulator
artificial
    breathing, a.

artificial *(continued)*
    palate, a.
    saliva, a.
    tears, a.
aryepiglottic (AE)
    cyst, a.
    fold, a.
    muscle, a.
aryepiglotticus
    muscle, a.
aryepiglottidean
arytenoepiglottic
arytenoid
    abduction, a.
    cartilage, a.
    eminence, a.
    process, a.
arytenoidectomy
arytenoideus
arytenoiditis
arytenoidopexy
AS (left ear)
Asai
    procedure, A.
    speech, A.
ascending ramus
Asch
    nasal splint, A.
    nasal-straightening forceps, A.
    operation, A.
    septal straightener, A.
    septal-straightening forceps, A.
Ascher syndrome
ascorbic acid
Asensio modification
Ash dental forceps
Asherson syndrome
asialia
asitia
asonia
aspergillosis
Aspergillus
    auricularis, A.
    niger, A.
    repens, A.
asphyxia

asphyxia *(continued)*
    carbonica, a.
    cyanotica, a.
    livida, a.
    local a.
    neonatorum, a.
    pallida, a.
    white a.
asphyxial
asphyxiant
asphyxiate
asphyxiation
aspirate
aspiration
    foreign body, a. of
    sinuses, a. of
aspirator
aspirin burn
Assezat triangle
associative aphasia
astemizole
asterion
asthenic habitus
asthma
    abdominal a.
    allergic a.
    alveolar a.
    atopic a.
    bacterial a.
    bronchial a.
    cardiac a.
    cat a.
    catarrhal a.
    Cheyne-Stokes a.
    convulsivum, a.
    cotton-dust a.
    cutaneous a.
    diisocyanate a.
    dust a.
    Elsner a.
    emphysematous a.
    essential a.
    extrinsic a.
    food a.
    grinders' a.
    Heberden a.

asthma *(continued)*
   horse a.
   humid a.
   infective a.
   intrinsic a.
   isocyanate a.
   Kopp a.
   Millar a.
   millers' a.
   miners' a.
   nasal a.
   nervous a.
   pollen a.
   potters' a.
   reflex a.
   Rostan a.
   sexual a.
   spasmodic a.
   steam-fitters' a.
   stone a.
   stripper's a.
   symptomatic a.
   thymic a.
   true a.
   Wichmann a.
asthma crystals
asthma paper
asthmatic
   bronchitis, a.
   cough, a.
asthmatiform
asthmatoid
   wheeze, a.
asthmogenic
asthmoid
   respiration, a.
astomia
astomus
atactic
ataxia
ataxic
   aphasia, a.
   nystagmus, a.
ataxophemia
atelectasis
atelectatic

atelocheilia
ateloglossia
atelognathia
ateloprosopia
atelostomia
Atkins-Tucker
   laryngoscope, A.
   shadow-free laryngoscope, A.
ATL (antitension lines)
atlantoaxial
atlantomastoid
atlanto-odontoid
atlas
atloido-occipital
atomizer
atopic
   allergy, a.
   asthma, a.
atopy
Atraloc needle
atresia
   aural a.
   esophageal a.
atresic
atretic
atretocephalus
atretolemia
atretorrhinia
atretostomia
atria (pl. of atrium)
atrium (pl. atria)
   glottidis, a.
   glottis, a. of
   laryngis, a.
   larynx, a. of
   matus medii, a.
atrophic
   catarrh, a.
   glossitis, a.
   laryngitis, a.
   pharyngitis, a.
   rhinitis, a.
attachment
   cuticle, a.
   epithelium, a.
attic

attic *(continued)*
    adhesion, a.
    disease, a.
    ear punch, a.
    middle ear, a. of
    perforation, a.
atticitis
atticoantral
atticoantrotomy
atticomastoid
atticotomy
    transmeatal a.
atticus
    punch, a.
attrahens
    aurem, a.
AU (both ears or each ear)
audibility
    curve, a.
    limit, a.
audible
    sound, a.
audile
audioanalgesia
audiogenic
audiogram
audiologist
audiology
audiometer
audiometric
audiometrician
audiometry
    averaged electroencephalic a.
    Bekesy a.
    cortical a.
    electrocochleographic a.
    electrodermal a.
    localization a.
    pure tone a.
    speech a.
AudioScope
audiosurgery
audiovisual
audiphone
audition
    chromatic a.

audition *(continued)*
    colored a.
    coloree, a.
    gustatory a.
    mental a.
auditive
auditognosis
audito-oculogyric reflex
auditory
    acuity, a.
    adaptation, a.
    aphasia, a.
    apparatus, a.
    area, a.
    aura, a.
    bulb, a.
    canal, a.
    cells, a.
    cortex, a.
    evoked response, a. (AER)
    meatus, a.
    muscles, a.
    nucleus, a.
    ossicle, a.
    pit, a.
    plate, a.
    reflex, a.
    sand, a.
    teeth of Huschke, a.
    tonsil of a. tube
    tube, a.
    W-22 test, a.
Aufricht
    rasp, A.
    retractor, A.
    sign, A.
    speculum, A.
Aufricht-Britetrace nasal retractor
Aufricht-Lipsett
    nasal rasp, A.
    raspatory, A.
augnathus
aura
    asthmatica, a.
aural
    nystagus, a.

aural *(continued)*
    vertigo, a.
Auralgan otic solution
aures (pl. of auris)
auricle
auricula (pl. auriculae)
    dextra, a.
    ear, a. of
    sinistra, a.
auriculae (pl. of auricula)
auricular
    arch, a.
    cartilage, a.
    ganglion, a.
    tubercle of Darwin, a.
auriculare
auricularis
auriculobregmatic
auriculocervical nerve reflex
auriculocranial
auriculo-occipital angle
auriculopalpebral reflex
auriculotemporal
auriculotherapy
auriculoventricular
auriform
aurilave
aurinarium
aurinasal
auriphone
auripuncture
auris (pl. aures)
    dextra, a. (AD)
    externa, a.
    interna, a.
    media, a.
    sinistra, a. (AS)
    uterque, a.
auriscalp
auriscalpium
auriscope
auriscopy
aurist
auristics
auristilla (pl. auristillae)
auristillae (pl. of auristilla)

aurogauge
aurometer
Austin
    dental knife, A.
    dental retractor, A.
    otological microsurgery set, A.
    strut calipers, A.
Austin-Shea tympanoplasty
autogenous graft
autograft
autolaryngoscope
autolaryngoscopy
automatic condenser
autophony
autoplasty
autopolymer resin
autospray
autotransplantation
autumnal catarrh
auxiliary abutment
Aveline Gutierrez parotidectomy
Avellis syndrome
averaged electroencephalic audiometry
aviation otitis
aviator's
    deafness, a.
    ear, a.
avulsed tooth
awl
axes (pl. of axis)
Axhausen cleft lip repair
axial
    angle, a.
    flap, a.
    line angle, a.
AxialTome
axiobuccal (AB)
axiobuccocervical (ABC)
axiobuccogingival (ABG)
axiobuccolingual (ABL)
axiocervical (AC)
axiodistal (AD)
axiodistocervical (ADC)
axiodistogingival (ADG)
axiodistoincisal (ADI)
axiodisto-occlusal (ADO)

axiogingival (AG)
axioincisal (AI)
axiolabial (ALA)
axiolabiogingival (ALAG)
axiolabiolingual (ALAL)
axiolingual (AL)
axiolinguocervical (ALC)
axiolinguogingival (ALG)
axiolinguo-occlusal (ALO)
axiomesial (AM)
axiomesiocervical (AMC)
axiomesiodistal (AMD)
axiomesiogingival (AMG)
axiomesioincisal (AMI)
axiomesio-occlusal (AMO)
axio-occlusal (AO)
axiopulpal (AP)
axipetal
axis (pl. axes)
   basibregmatic a.
   basicranial a.
   basifacial a.
   binauricular a.

axis (pl. axes) *(continued)*
   condylar a.
   craniofacial a.
   Downs Y a.
   facial a.
   frontal a.
   hinge a.
   mandibular a.
   opening a.
   optical a.
   preparation, a. of
   thyroid a.
   visual a.
   Y a.
axis ligament
axoneme
axonotmesis
axoplasm
Ayerza disease
Aztec ear
azygoesophageal
   recess, a.

Additional entries

B

B12 dental curette
B (buccal)
BA (buccoaxial)
Babbitt metal
Babcock-Lindemann ostectomy
Babinski-Weil test
baby tooth
BABYbird infant respirator
BAC (buccoaxiocervical)
Bacitracin
back-biting forceps
backward caries
bactericidal
bactericide
bacteriostatic
Bacteroides
bad breath
Baelz disease
Baer plane
Bafverstadt syndrome
BAG (buccoaxiogingival)
bag
    Politzer b.
bagged
bagging
baggy eyes
Bakamjian deltopectoral flap
baked tongue
Baker
    anchorage, B.
    bar, B.
    formula, B.
    syndrome, B.
    velum, B.
BAL (bronchoalveolar lavage)
balanced bite
balancing contact
balcony lingual procedure
bald tongue
ball burnisher
Ball elevator
Ballenger
    bur, B.

Ballenger *(continued)*
    curette, B.
    elevator, B.
    ethmoid curette, B.
    follicle electrode, B.
    forceps, B.
    gouge, B.
    mastoid bur, B.
    nose knife, B.
    swivel knife, B.
    tonsil forceps, B.
Ballenger-Hajek
    chisel, B.
    elevator, B.
Ballenger-Lillie mastoid bur
Ballenger-Sluder
    guillotine, B.
    tonsillectome, B.
balloon
    intranasal b.
balloon dilatation
balloon nasostat
ballooning
    esophagoscope, b.
    sella turcica, b. of
balm of Gilead
Balme cough
balsam of Gilead
Baltimore nasal scissors
band
    anchor b.
    clamp b.
    contoured b.
    elastic b.
    matrix b.
    molar b.
    orthodontic b.
    phonatory b's
banding
Bane forceps
bank
    skin b.
    tissue b.

bar
   arch b.
   connector b.
   dental b.
   Erich arch b.
   hyoid b.
   Kazanjian T b.
   Kennedy b.
   labial b.
   lingual b.
   occlusal rest b.
   palatal b.
   Passavant's b.
bar clasp arm
Barany
   symptom, B.
   syndrome, B.
   test, B.
barbed broach
Barber
   needle, B.
   pick, B.
Bard-Parker (B-P)
   knife, B.
   U-Mid/Lo humidifier, B.
Bardach modification of Obwegeser mandibular osteotomy procedure
barium
   swallow, b.
   test, b.
Barker point
barking cough
Barlow forceps
Barnhill curette
barodontalgia
baro-otitis
   media, b.
Baron
   ear knife, B.
   ear tube, B.
   palate elevator, B.
barosinusitis
barotitis
   media, b.
barotrauma
   otitic b.

barotrauma *(continued)*
   sinus b.
Barrett
   epithelium, B.
   esophagus, B.
   ulcer, B.
Barsky
   cleft lip repair, B.
   elevator, B.
   osteotome, B.
   otoplasty, B.
   pharyngoplasty, B.
Barth
   mastoid curette, B.
   mastoid knife, B.
Bartholin duct
bartholinitis
Barton dressing
baryglossia
barylalia
baryphonia
basal
   cell cancer, b.
   lamina, b.
   neck fracture, b.
   olfactory bundle of Wallenburg, b.
   ridge, b.
   seat, b.
   seat area, b.
basalar prognathism
basaloid mixed tumor
base
   acrylic resin b.
   apical b.
   cavity b.
   cement b.
   denture b.
   metal b.
   plastic b.
   record b.
   shellac b's
   stapes, b. of
   temporary b.
   tinted denture b.
   tooth-borne b.
   trial b.

Basedow goiter
baseline
baseplate
    gutta-percha b.
    stabilized b.
baseplate wax
bases (pl. of basis)
basial
basialis
basialveolar
basibregmatic axis
basicranial axis
basifacial axis
basihyal
basihyoid
basilar
    crest, b.
    fracture, b.
basilaris
    cranii, b.
basinasial
basioccipital
basioglossus
basion
basirhinal
basis (pl. bases)
basisphenoid
basitemporal
basket crown
bass deafness
bat ear
Battle
    operation, B.
    sign, B.
batwing incision
Bauer-Tondra-Trusler cleft lip repair
Bauer-Trusler-Tondra cleft lip repair
Bauhin gland
Baum tonsil needle holder
Baum-Hecht tarsorrhaphy forceps
bayonet saw
Bazex syndrome
BC (bone conduction or buccocervical)
BD (buccodistal)
Bead ethmoid forceps
beaked nose

beaker cell
BEAR cub ventilator
BEAR I adult volume ventilator
bearing
    central b.
Beardsley esophageal retractor
beaten silver appearance
Beaver
    handle, B.
    myringotomy blade, B.
    tonsillectomy blade, B.
bechic
Bechterev
    nucleus, B.
    reflex, B.
Bechterew
    nucleus, B.
    reflex, B.
Beck Depression Inventory
Beck-Mueller tonsillectome
Beck-Schenck tonsillectome
Beck-Storz tonsil snare
Becker otoplasty
Beckman
    nasal scissors, B.
    nasal speculum, B.
Beckman-Colver nasal speculum
Beclard triangle
beclomethasone dipropionate
Bednar aphthae
beefy
    -red mucosa, b.
    tongue, b.
beeswax
Begg appliance
begma
Behcet syndrome
Bekesy audiometry
Bekhterev
    nucleus, B,
    reflex, B.
bel
belching
Bell
    palsy, B.
    procedure, B.

Bell *(continued)*
  spasm, B.
Bellocq cannula
Bellucci
  ear scissors, B.
  nasal suction tube, B.
  otolaryngology scissors, B.
Belsey
  esophagoplasty, B.
  Mark IV operation, B.
Belz lacrimal sac rongeur
Benadryl
benign migratory glossitis
Benjamin
  binocular slimline laryngoscope, B.
  pediatric laryngoscope, B.
Benjamin-Havas fiberoptic light clip
Bennett
  angle, B.
  movement, B.
Bennett ventilator
Beneys tonsil compressor
benzoin
Beraud valve
Berci-Ward laryngopharyngoscope
Berens thyroid retractor
Bergh cilia forceps
Berke operation
  operation, B.
  ptosis clamp, b.
Berke-Motais technique
Berman
  disposable airway, B.
  intubating pharyngeal airway, B.
Bermingham nasal douche
Bern
  forceps, B.
  rasp, B.
Bernard-Burrows procedure
Bernay
  sponge, B.
  tracheal retractor, B.
Berne
  nasal forceps, B.
  nasal rasp, B.
  nasal raspatory, B.

Bernstein test
Berry ligament
Bertel position
Bertin bone
Beschet hiatus
Besey esophagram
Bespaloff sign
beta-hemolytic
betel leaf
bevel
beveled
beveling
Beyer
  atticus punch, b.
  forceps, B.
  rongeur, B.
Bezold
  abscess, B.
  ganglion, B.
  mastoiditis, B.
  perforation, B.
  triad, B.
Bezold-Edelman tuning fork
BF large-core bronchoscope
BG (buccogingival)
biarticular
biauricular
bibeveled
bicameral
Bickel ring
biconcave
biconvex
bicuspid tooth
bicuspidal
bicuspidate
bicuspidization
bicuspoid
bidental
bidentate
Biderman sign
Bieg sign
bifacial
bifid
  tongue, b.
  uvula, b.
bigonial diameter

bile reflux
Billeau
    ear curette. B.
    ear knife, B.
    ear loop, B.
Billroth procedure
bilobed flap
bilophont
bimastoid
bimaxillary
    dentoalveolar protrusion, b.
    protrusion, b.
bimeter gnathodynamometer
Bimler
    activator, B.
    appliance, B.
binangle
binasal pharyngeal airway
binaural
    distorted speech test, b.
    stethoscope, b.
binauricular axis
Bing test
Binnie otoplasty
binophthalmoscope
binotic
biocompatible
Biocoral
Bio-EMG 800
Biofinisher
biomaterial
biomechanics
biophysics
Biot breathing
Bi-OX III ear oximeter
biparietal diameter
Bipro orthodontic appliance
Bird
    Asthmastik, B.
    humidifier, B.
    machine, B.
    respirator, B.
bird-beak
    distal esophagus, b.
    jaw, b.
bird-face deformity

biscuit
biscuiting
Bishop
    antrum trocar, B.
    chisel, B.
    mastoid gouge, B.
bismuth
    gingivitis, b.
    line, b.
    stomatitis, b.
bisque
bistoury
    ear b.
    nasal b.
    tracheal b.
bistoury blade
bistoury knife
bite
    balanced b.
    check b.
    close b.
    closed b.
    cross b.
    deep b.
    edge-to-edge b.
    end-to-end b.
    open b.
    over b.
    scissors b.
    underhung b.
    wax b.
    X-b.
bite-block
    fixed turban, b.
    on a stick, b.
bite gauge
bite line
bite rim
bite splint
bitegage
bitelock
bitemporal diameter
biteplane
biteplate
bite-wing radiograph
biting forceps

bivalved ear speculum
bivalving incision
Bivona
   low-resistance voice prosthesis, B.
   tracheostomy tube, B.
   voice prosthesis, B.
bizygomatic
   breadth, b.
   diameter, b.
Bizzari-Guiffrida
   knife, B.
   laryngoscope, B.
Bjornstad syndrome
BL (buccolingual)
BLA (buccolabial)
black
   copper cement, b.
   hairy tongue, b.
   measles, b.
   tongue, b.
Black classification
Blade-Wilde ear forceps
Blainville ear
Blair
   cleft palate clamp, B.
   cleft palate elevator, B.
   cleft palate knife, B.
   head drape, B.
   incision, B.
   ptosis correction procedure, B.
Blair-Brown
   graft, B.
   operation, B.
Blake
   disk, B.
   ear forceps, B.
   esophageal tube, B.
Blakemore esophageal tube
Blakemore-Sengstaken tube
Blakesley
   ethmoid forceps, B.
   lacrimal trephine, B.
   septal compression forceps, B.
   tongue depressor, B.
   uvula retractor, B.
Blakesley-Wilde

Blakesley-Wilde *(continued)*
   ear forceps, B.
   ethmoid forceps, B.
Blandin
   ganglion, B.
   glands, B.
Blandin and Nuhn glands
Blasius duct
Blaskovics operation
bleaching
bleb
bleeder
bleeding
   diathesis, b.
   esophageal varices, b.
   gums, b.
   point, b.
   site, b.
blennadenitis
blennogenic
blennogenous
blennoid
blennorrhagia
blennorrhea
   Stoerk b.
blennostasis
blennostatic
blepharadenitis
blepharectomy
blepharitis
blepharoadenoma
blepharoatheroma
blepharochalasis
blepharodiastasis
blepharoncus
blepharopachynsis
blepharophimosis
blepharoplasty
blepharoplegia
blepharoptosis
blepharorrhaphy
blepharospasm
blepharosphincterectomy
blepharosynechia
blepharotomy
blind

blind *(continued)*
    abscess, b.
    osteotomy, b.
    pit, b.
    sight, b.
    spot, b.
    upper esophageal pouch, b.
blindness
block
    ear b.
    intranasal b.
    sinus b.
blocked
    airway, b.
    breathing passage, b.
    nasal passage, b.
blockout
    wax, b.
Blocksma technique
Blohmka
    tonsil forceps, B.
    tonsil hemostat, B.
Blom-Singer
    duckbill voice prosthesis, B.
    postlaryngectomy valve, B.
    tracheoesophageal fistula, B.
    vocal reconstruction, B.
    voice valve, B.
blood
    -brain barrier, b.
    C&S, b.
    culture, b.
    culture and sensitivity, b.
Blount brace
blow-in fracture
blow-out fracture
blue
    asphyxia, b.
    baby, b.
    bloater, b.
    gum, b.
    line, b.
    Shepard grommet tube, b.
Blum technique
Blumenbach
    clivus, B.

Blumenbach *(continued)*
    plane, B.
    process, B.
blunt
    dissection, b.
    dissection and snare method, b.
    dissector, b.
blush
BM (buccomesial)
BMS (burning mouth syndrome)
BNPA (binasal pharyngeal airway)
BO (bucco-occlusal)
Bochdalek ganglion
Bockenheimer-Axhausen procedure
Bock nerve
Boerhaave syndrome
Boettcher
    forceps, B.
    hook. B.
    scissors, B.
    tonsil artery forceps, B.
    tonsil hook, B.
Boettcher-Farlow snare
Boettcher-Jennings gag
Boettcher-Schnidt antrum trocar
bogginess
boggy
Bohn
    nodules, B.
    pearls, B.
Boies
    cutting forceps, B.
    nasal fracture elevator, B.
Boiler septal trephine
boilermaker's deafness
Boilo
    head mirror, B.
    laryngeal mirror, B.
Boitel bar
Boley gauge
Bolton
    -nasion plane, B.
    point, B.
    triangle, B.
bolus
    alimentary b.

bolus *(continued)*
    food b.
bolus stent
bolused
BOM (bilateral otitis media)
bonding
    tooth b.
Bondy mastoidectomy
bone
    ash, b.
    -biting forceps, b.
    chip, b.
    chisel, b.
    conduction, b. (BC)
    dust, b.
    hyoid b.
    paté, b.
    petrous b.
    plate, b.
    slurry, b.
    squamosal b.
    temporal b.
    tympanic b.
    zygomatic b.
Bonwill
    crown, B.
    triangle, B.
bony
    attachment, b.
    bridge, b.
    chain, b.
    crypt, b.
    hard palate, b.
    hump, b.
    labyrinth, b.
    landmarks, b.
    palate, b.
    spicule, b.
    spur, b.
Boo-Chai classification
Book syndrome
border
    alveolar b. of mandible
    alveolar b. of maxilla
    denture b.
    inferior b. of mandible

border *(continued)*
    orbital b. of sphenoid bone
    vermilion b.
border movement
Bordetella parapertussis
Borjeson syndrome
Borjeson-Forssman-Lehmann syndrome
Boros esophagoscope
Bose
    tracheal hook, B.
    tracheotomy, B.
Bosker TMI system
boss
bosselated
bosselation
Bostock catarrh
Boston exanthem
Bosworth
    headband, B.
    nasal saw, B.
    nasal snare, B.
    Super-EBA cement, B.
    tongue depressor, B.
bottle mouth caries
bouche
    de tapir, b.
Bouchut tubes
bougie
    Hurst b's
    Maloney b's
bougienage
Bourns
    BEAR I ventilator, B.
    humidifier, B.
bouquet
bovine
    face, b.
    facies, b.
    fascia graft, b.
bow
    face b
    Logan b.
bow activator
Bowman
    probe, B.
    glands, B.

Box adenotome
Box-DeJager adenotome
boxing
   wax, b.
Boyce sign
Boyer
   bursa, B.
   cyst, B.
Boyle law
Boyle-Davis mouth gag
Boyne dental prosthesis
BP (buccopulpal)
B-P (Bard-Parker)
brace
   Blount b.
brachiofaciolingual
brachycheilia
brachyesophagus
brachyfacial
brachygnathia
brachygnathous
brachystaphyline
bracket
bracketed
Brackett dental probe
Bradford
   thyroid forceps, B.
   thyroid traction vulsellum forceps, B.
bradyacusia
bradyecoia
bradyglossia
bradylalia
bradylogia
bradyphagia
bradyphasia
bradyphemia
bradyphrasia
Brailey stretching of supratrochlear nerve
brain
   hernia, b.
   stem, b.
branchial
   arch, b.
   cartilage, b.
   cleft, b.
   cleft sinusectomy, b.

branchial *(continued)*
   duct, b.
   fistula, b.
   grooves, b.
   muscles, b.
   pouch, b.
   sinus, b.
branchiogenic
branchiogenous
branchioma
branchiomere
branchiomeric
branchiomerism
Branhamella
   catarrhalis, B.
brass poisoning
brassy cough
Brauer procedure
Braun graft
Braun-Wangensteen graft
Brawley
   antrum rasp, B.
   frontal sinus rasp, B.
   nasal suction tip, B.
Brazilian blastomycosis
breadth
   bizygomatic b.
   finger-b.
breath
   sounds, b.
breathe
breathiness
breathing
bredouillement
bregma
   -menton film, b.
Breitman adenotome
Brenner formula
Brent pressure earring
Breschet sinus
Bresgen sinus probe
Breslow classification
Brethaire
Bretonneau diphtheria
brevicollis
Brewster sinus punch

Brickner sign
bridge
    cantilever b.
    dental b.
    dentin b.
    extension b.
    fixed b.
    fixed b. with rigid connectors
    fixed b. with rigid and nonrigid connectors
    fixed-fixed b.
    fixed-movable b.
    nose, b. of
    removable b.
    stationary b.
bridge impression
bridgework
    fixed b.
    removable b.
Briggs laryngoscope
Brighton epistaxis balloon
bristle cells
Bristow zygomatic elevator
broach
    barbed b.
    pathfinder b.
    root canal b.
    smooth b.
Broadbent registration point
Broadbent-Bolton plane
broad-spectrum coverage
Broca
    angle, B.
    aphasia, B.
    motor speech area, B.
    parolfactory area, B.
    point, B.
Brompton cocktail
bronch (bronchoscopy)
bronchadenitis
bronched (bronchoscopy was performed)
bronchi (4th, 5th, 6th order) (pl. of bronchus)
bronchia (pl. of bronchium)
bronchial
    antispasmodic, b.

bronchial *(continued)*
    asthma, b.
    atresia, b.
    breath sounds, b.
    breathing, b.
    brush biopsy, b.
    brushing, b.
    bud, b.
    calculus, b.
    cartilage, b.
    check-valve, b.
    cough, b.
    crisis, b.
    drainage, b.
    fremitus, b.
    glands, b.
    lavage, b.
    markings, b.
    mucus blanket, b.
    mucus inhibitor, b.
    rales, b.
    rupture, b.
    secretions, b.
    spasm, b.
    tree, b.
    tube, b.
    washings, b.
    wheezing, b.
bronchiectasis
    capillary b.
    cylindrical b.
    cystic b.
    dry b.
    follicular b.
    saccular b.
bronchiectatic
    collapse, b.
bronchiloquy
bronchiocele
bronchiocrisis
bronchiolar
bronchiole
bronchiolectasis
bronchioli (pl. of bronchiolus)
bronchiolitis
    acute obliterating b.

bronchiolitis *(continued)*
    exudativa, b.
    fibrosa obliterans, b.
    vesicular b.
bronchiolus (pl. bronchioli)
bronchiospasm
bronchiostenosis
bronchismus
bronchitic
bronchitis
    acute b.
    acute laryngotracheal b.
    arachidic b.
    asthmatic b.
    capillary b.
    Castellani b.
    catarrhal b.
    cheesy b.
    chronic b.
    croupous b.
    dry b.
    ether b.
    exudative b.
    fibrinous b.
    hemorrhagic b.
    infectious asthmatic b.
    mechanic b.
    membranous b.
    obliterans, b.
    phthinoid b.
    plastic b.
    productive b.
    pseudomembranous b.
    putrid b.
    secondary b.
    staphyloccus b.
    streptococcal b.
    suffocative b.
    vegetal b.
    vesicular b.
bronchiolitis
    obliterans, b.
bronchium (pl. bronchia)
bronchoadenitis
bronchoalveolar
    lavage, b. (BAL)

bronchoalveolar *(continued)*
    lavage fluid, b. (BALF)
    washings, b.
bronchoalveolitis
bronchoaspergillosis
bronchoblastomycosis
bronchoblennorrhea
bronchocandidiasis
Broncho-Cath endotracheal tube
bronchocavernous
bronchocele
bronchoconstriction
bronchoconstrictor
bronchodilatation
bronchodilation
bronchodilator
bronchoedema
bronchoegophony
bronchoesophageal
bronchoesophagoscope
bronchoesophagoscopy
bronchofiberscope
bronchofiberscopy
bronchogenic
bronchogram
    air b.
bronchography
    Cope-method b.
    inhalation b.
    percutaneous transtracheal b.
broncholith
broncholithiasis
bronchomalacia
bronchomoniliasis
bronchomotor
bronchomucotropic
bronchomycosis
bronchonocardiosis
broncho-oidiosis
bronchopathy
bronchophony
    pectoriloquous b.
    sniffling b.
    whispered b.
bronchoplasty
bronchoplegia

bronchopneumonia
bronchopulmonary
bronchorrhagia
bronchorrhea
bronchorrhoncus
bronchoscope
   fiberoptic b.
bronchoscope aspirating tube
bronchoscope battery box
bronchoscopic
   bougie, b.
   brush, b.
   cleaning tool, b.
   face shield, b.
   magnet, b.
   rule, b.
   telescope, b.
bronchoscopy
   fiberoptic b.
bronchosinusitis
bronchospasm
bronchospastic
   component, b.
bronchospirochetosis
bronchospirography
bronchospirometer
bronchospirometric
   catheter, b.
bronchospirometry
bronchostaxis
bronchostenosis
bronchostomy
bronchotome
bronchotomy
bronchotracheal
   aspirate, b.
   aspiration, b.
bronchovesicular
bronchus (pl. bronchi)
Bronkaid Mist
Bronkometer
Bronkosol
Brophy
   bistoury knife, B.
   cleft palate knife, B.
   cleft palate operation, B.

Brophy *(continued)*
   mouth gag, B.
   plate, B.
Broviac catheter
brow
brown
   mixture, b.
   pellicle, b.
   teeth, b.
   tumor, b.
Brown
   cleft palate knife, B.
   dermatome, B.
   ear speculum, B.
   nasal applicator, B.
   nasal splint, B.
   needle, B.
   pushback palatoplasty, B.
   snare, B.
   staphylorrhaphy needle, B.
   tonsillectome, B.
   tonsil snare, B.
Brown-Adson forceps
Brown-Blair procedure
Brown-Davis gag
Brown-Fryer-MacDowell procedure
Brown-McHardy pneumatic dilator
Broyles
   anterior commissure laryngoscope, B.
   bronchoscope, B.
   dilator, B.
   esophageal dilator, B.
   esophagoscope, B.
   laryngoscope, B.
   nasopharyngoscope, B.
   telescope, B.
Bruce tract
Bruch mastoid retractor
Brudzinski sign
Bruening
   ear snare, B.
   electroscope, B.
   esophagoscope, B.
   ethmoid exenteration forceps, B.
   forceps, B.
   nasal-cutting septum forceps, B.

Bruening *(continued)*
    nasal snare, B.
    otoscope, B.
    punch, B.
    snare, B.
Brun
    ear curette, B.
    mastoid curette, B.
Brunn membrane
Brunner goiter dissector
Brunton otoscope
brushing
brusque dilatation of esophagus
brux
bruxism
bruxomania
Bryant nasal forceps
BTE (behind the ear)
bubble humidifier
bucca
    cavi oris, b.
buccal (B)
    angles, b.
    cavity, b.
    crossbite, b.
    curve, b.
    fat pad, b.
    gingiva, b.
    gland, b.
    gutter, b.
    lymph node, b.
    mucosa, b.
    pedicle flap, b.
    smear, b.
    tablet, b.
    tooth, b.
    tube, b.
buccally
buccinatolabialis
buccinator
    crest, b.
    lymph node, b.
    muscle, b.
buccoaxial (BA)
buccoaxiocervical (BAC)
buccoaxiogingival (BAG)

buccocervical (BC)
buccoclusal
buccoclusion
buccodistal (BD)
buccogingival (BG)
buccoglossopharyngitis
    sicca, b.
buccolabial (BLA)
buccolingual (BL)
    diameter, b.
buccomaxillary
buccomesial (BM)
bucconasal
bucco-occlusal (BO)
buccopharyngeal
buccoplacement
buccopulpal (BP)
buccoversion
buccula
Buck
    curette, B.
    ear applicator, B.
    ear knife, B.
    mastoid curette, B
    myringotome, B.
    myringotomy knife, B.
    nasal applicator, B.
buck teeth
bucket-handle view of nasal bones
bud
    bronchial b.
    gustatory b.
    lung b.
    taste b.
    tooth b.
Budin joint
Budinger blepharoplasty
building solder
bulb
    auditory b.
    gustatory b.
    olfactory b.
bulbous
    tip, b.
bulbus
    oculi, b.

bulbus *(continued)*
   olfactorius, b.
bulimia
   nervosa, b.
bulimic
bulimorexia
bull neck
bulla (pl. bullae)
   ethmoid b.
   ethmoidalis cavi nasi, b.
   ethmoidalis ossis ethmoidalis, b.
   mastoidea, b.
   ossea, b.
bullae (pl. of bulla)
bulldog nasal scissors
bullous
   myringitis, b.
bunodont
bunolophodont
bunoselenodont
bur
   diamond b.
bur hole
buried tonsil
Burkitt lymphoma
burning
   mouth syndrome, b. (BMS)
   tongue, b.
burnish
burnisher
burnishing
burnout wax
Burns space
Burow
   blepharoplasty, B.
   solution, B.
   triangle procedure, B.
burred
Burrow triangle
bursa (pl. bursae)
   Boyer b.

bursa (pl. bursae) *(continued)*
   Calori b.
   Fleischmann b.
   hyoid b.
   infrahyoid b.
   Luschka b.
   pharyngea, b.
   pharyngeal b.
   retrohyoid b.
   sternohyoid b.
   subcutanea prominentiae
      laryngeaalis, b.
   subcutaneous b. of prominence of
      larynx
   subhyoid b.
   tensor veli palatini muscle, b. of
   Thornwaldt b.
   thyrohyoid b.
   Tornwaldt b.
bursae (pl. of bursa)
bursitis
   pharyngeal b.
   Thornwaldt b.
   Tornwaldt b.
bursolith
Burton laryngoscope
Butler
   dental retractor, B.
   ear forceps, B.
   tonsil suction tube, B.
butterfly
   incision, b.
   rash, b.
button
   collar b.
   tracheostomy, b.
buttonhole
   fracture, b.
buttress
buttressed

C

cachectic
    aphthae, c.
cachexia
cacogeusia
cacosmia
Caffey disease
Cagot ear
calcic
    ulatrophy, c.
calciprivia
calcitite bone graft
calcium
    hydroxide cement, c.
calculi (pl. of calculus)
calculus (pl. calculi)
    bronchial c.
    dental c.
    lacrimal c.
    nasal c.
    salivary c.
    subgingival c.
    supragingival c.
    tonsillar c.
Caldwell
    position, C.
    view, C.
Caldwell-Luc
    incision, C.
    operation, C.
    window procedure, C.
Calgiswab
caliber
calibrate
calibration
calibrator
caliculi (pl. of caliculus)
caliculus (pl. caliculi)
    gustatorius, c.
caliper
    skinfold c.
Callahan method
Calleja islands
Calori bursa

caloric
    nystagmus, c.
    test, c.
calyculus
    gustatorius, c.
CAM (Child Adult Mist) Tent
Camille Bernard lip repair
Campe procedure
camphor
camphorated oil
canal
    accessory palatine c's
    alisphenoid c.
    alveolar c.
    Arnold c.
    auditory c.
    bony c's of ear
    caroticotympanic c's
    carotid c.
    chorda tympani, c. of
    cochlear c.
    condylar c.
    condyloid c.
    Corti, c. of
    Cotunnius, c. of
    craniopharyngeal c.
    crural c.
    crural c. of Henle
    dental c's
    dentinal c's
    Dorello c.
    ethmoidal c.
    eustachian c.
    external auditory c.
    facial c.
    fallopian c.
    Ferrein c.
    Guidi, c. of
    Hirschfeld c's
    His c.
    Huschke c.
    hypoglossal c.
    incisal c.

canal *(continued)*
    incisive c.
    infraorbital c.
    interdental c's
    interfacial c's
    Jacobson c.
    Lowenberg c.
    mandibular c.
    maxillary c.
    nasal c.
    nasolacrimal c.
    nasopalatine c.
    olfactory c.
    palatine c.
    palatomaxillary c.
    palatovaginal c.
    petromastoid c.
    pharyngeal c.
    pterygoid c.
    pterygopalatine c.
    pulp c.
    Rivinus, c. of
    root c.
    Rosenthal c.
    sacculocochlear c.
    sacculoutricular c.
    semicircular c's
    sphenopalatine c.
    sphenopharyngeal c.
    sphenopterygoid c.
    spiral c.
    spiroid c.
    Steno, c. of
    Stensen c.
    supraciliary c.
    supraoptic c.
    supraorbital c.
    tensor tympani, c.
    Tourtual c.
    tubal c.
    tubotympanic c.
    tympanic c. of cochlea
    utriculosaccular c.
    vestibular c.
    vomerine c.
    vomerobasilar c.

canal *(continued)*
    vomerorostral c.
    vomerovaginal c.
    zygomaticofacial c.
    zygomaticotemporal c.
canales (pl. of canalis)
canalicular
canaliculi (pl. of canaliculus)
canaliculitis
canaliculization
canaliculodacryocystostomy
canaliculorhinostomy
canaliculus (pl. canaliculi)
    caroticotympanic c's
    chorda tympani, c. of
    cochlea, c. of
    dental c's
    incisor c.
    lacrimalis, c.
    mastoid c.
    mastoid c. for Arnold nerve
    mastoideus, c.
    tympanic c.
    tympanic c. for Jacobson nerve
    tympanicus, c.
canaliculus punch
canalis (pl. canales)
    basipharyngeus, c.
    caroticus, c.
    chordae tympani, c.
    condylaris, c.
    condyloideus, c.
    facialis, c.
    hypoglossalis, c.
    incisivus, c.
    infraorbitalis, c.
    mandibulae, c.
    musculotubarius, c.
    nasolacrimalis, c.
    palatinus, c.
    palatovaginalis, c.
    pharyngeus, c.
    pterygoideus, c.
    pterygopalatinus, c.
    radicis dentis, c.
    semicircularis, c.

canalis (pl. canales) *(continued)*
   spiralis cochleae, c.
   spiralis modioli, c.
   vomerostralis, c.
   vomerovaginalis, c.
canalization
canaloplasty
canal knife
canal skin
canal wall
cancrum
   nasi, c.
   oris, c.
Candida
   albicans, C.
candidiasis
Canfield
   knife, C.
   procedure, C.
canine
   eminence, c.
   fossa, c.
   spasm, c.
   tooth, c.
   -to-canine lingual splint, c.
caninus
canker sore
cannula (pl. cannulae)
cannulae (pl. of cannula)
cannulate
cannulization
cant of mandible
canthal
canthectomy
canthi (pl. of canthus)
canthitis
cantholysis
canthomeatal
   flap, c.
   line, c.
canthoplasty
canthorrhaphy
canthotomy
canthus (pl. canthi)
cantilever bridge
cantus galli

cap
   enamel c.
   tooth c.
cap crown
cap splint
capillary
   bronchitis, c.
   fracture, c.
capita (pl. of caput)
capitula (pl. of capitulum)
capitulum (pl. capitula)
   mallei, c.
   mandibulae, c.
   stapedis, c.
   stapes, c. of.
capped teeth
capping
   pulp c.
capriloquism
capsula (pl. capsulae)
capsulae (pl. of capsula)
capsular
capsule
   auditory c.
   nasal c.
   optic c.
   otic c.
   temporomandibular joint c.
   tonsil, c. of
   tonsillar c.
capsulopalpebral
caput (pl. capita)
   progeneum, c.
   stapedis, c.
Carabelli
   cusp, C.
   sign, C.
   tubercle, C.
carbachol
carbide mastoid bur
carbolfuchsin stain
carbonaceous
Carborundum disk
carcinoma
carcinomatous
cardinal tongue

carding wax
cardioesophageal
 junction, c.
 sphincter, c.
Carhart
 notch, C.
 tone decay test, C.
caries
 arrested c.
 backward c.
 bottle mouth c.
 cemental c.
 central c.
 dental c.
 dentinal c.
 dry c.
 enamel c.
 fungosa, c.
 internal c.
 lateral c.
 necrotic c.
 pit c.
 radiation c.
 rampant c.
 sicca, c.
carina (pl. carinae)
 nasi, c.
 trachea, c. of
 tracheae, c.
carinae (pl. of carina)
cariogenesis
cariogenic
cariogenicity
cariology
cariosity
carious
 teeth, c.
Carlens double-lumen endotracheal tube
C-arm fluoroscopy
Carmack curette
Carmalt clamp
Carmody-Batson
 approach, C.
 procedure, C.
caroticotympanic canals
carotid

carotid *(continued)*
 arch, c.
 artery, c.
 bruit, c.
 canal, c.
 massage, c.
 sheath, c.
 triangle, c.
carotidynia
Carpenter tonsil knife
carpopedal spasm
Carpue rhinoplasty
carpule
Carter
 intranasal splint, C.
 operation, C.
cartilage
 accessory c's of nose
 alar c.
 arytenoid c.
 auditory tube, c. of
 auricular c.
 branchial c.
 conchal c.
 corniculate c.
 cricoid c.
 cuneiform c.
 dentinal c.
 epactal c's
 epiglottic c.
 eustachian c.
 gingival c.
 guttural c.
 hyaline c.
 intrathyroid c.
 laryngeal c. of Luschka
 Luschka c.
 mandibular c.
 meatal c.
 minor c's
 nasal c.
 periotic c.
 posterior cricoarytenoid c.
 pyramidal c.
 Reichert c.
 Santorini, c. of

cartilage *(continued)*
    scutiform c.
    septal c. of nose
    sesamoid c.
    subvomerine c.
    supra-arytenoid c.
    thyroid c.
    tracheal c.
    triangular c. of nose
    triquetral c.
    tubal c.
    tympanomandibular c.
    vomeronasal c.
    Wrisberg, c. of
cartilage graft
cartilagines (pl. of cartilago)
    alares minores, c.
    laryngis, c.
    nasales accessoriae, c.
    nasi, c.
    sesamoideae nasi, c.
    tracheales, c.
cartilaginous
    hump, c.
    ring, c.
    septum, c.
    vault, c.
cartilago (pl. cartilagines)
    alaris major, c.
    arytenoidea, c.
    auriculae, c.
    corniculata, c.
    cricoidea, c.
    cuneiformis c.
    epiglottica, c.
    jacobsoni, c.
    laryngis, c.
    meatus acustici, c.
    nasi lateralis, c.
    santorini, c.
    septi nasi, c.
    sesamoidea laryngis c.
    sesamoidea ligamenti vocalis, c.
    thyroidea, c.
    triquetra c.
    tubae auditivae, c.

cartilago (pl. cartilagines) *(continued)*
    vomeronasalis, c.
    wrisbergi, c.
cartilaginous
    ring, c.
caruncle
    lacrimal c.
    sublingual c.
caruncula
    salivaris, c.
    sublingualis, c.
carver
    amalgam c.
    wax c.
Casal necklace
caseation
caseous
    abscess, c.
    tonsillitis, c.
Cassel procedure
Casselberry
    position, C.
    sphenoid washing tube, C.
Casser ligament
casserian ligament
cast
    dental c.
    diagnostic c.
    gnathostatic c.
    investment c.
    master c.
    preextraction c.
    preoperative c.
    refractory c.
    study c.
cast core
cast splint
Castanares
    bilateral blepharoplasty, C.
    face-lift scissors, C.
Castellani bronchitis
Castelli tube
Castelli-Paparella
    collar-button tube, C.
    myringotomy tube, C.
casting

casting *(continued)*
    flask, c.
    wax, c.
cat
    asthma, c.
    -scratch disease, c.
    -scratch fever, c.
catarrh
    atrophic c.
    autumnal c.
    Bostock c.
    dry c.
    hypertrophic c.
    Laennec c.
    postnasal c.
    sinus c.
    suffocative c.
catarrhal
    asthma, c.
    bronchitis, c.
    croup, c.
    gingivitis, c.
    mastoiditis, c.
    pharyngitis, c.
    stomatitis, c.
catarrhine
caterpillaring
cauda
    helicus, c.
caudal
cauliflower ear
Caulk Nuva-Tach
causalgia
Causse piston
cauterization
cauterize
cautery
cava (pl. of cavum)
Cavanaugh-Wells tonsil forceps
cavernous sinus
    thrombosis, c.
Cavit seal
cavitas (pl. cavitates)
    conchae, c.
    coronalis, c.
    dentis, c.

cavitas (pl. cavitates) *(continued)*
    infraglottica, c.
    laryngis, c.
    nasi, c.
    oris, c.
    pharyngis, c.
    pulparis, c.
    tympanica, c.
cavitates (pl. of cavitas)
cavitation
Cavitron dental unit
cavity
    alveolar c.
    bony c. of nose
    buccal c.
    complex c.
    compound c.
    concha, c. of
    dental c.
    distal c.
    faucial c.
    fissure c.
    incisal c.
    infraglottic c.
    labial c.
    laryngeal c.
    laryngopharyngeal c.
    lingual c.
    mastoid c.
    mesial c.
    nasal c.
    nerve c.
    occlusal c.
    oral c.
    pharyngeal c.
    pharyngolaryngeal c.
    pharyngonasal c.
    pharyngo-oral c.
    pit c.
    prepared c.
    proximal c.
    pulp c.
    Rosenmuller c.
    simple c.
    tympanic c.
cavity angles

cavity base
cavity classification
cavity liner
cavity preparation
cavity varnish
cavography
cavosurface angle
cavum (pl. cava)
   conchae, c.
   conchum, c.
   infraglotticum, c.
   laryngis, c.
   nasi, c.
   nasi osseum, c.
   oris, c.
   oris externum, c.
   pharyngis, c.
   tympani, c.
Cawthorne
   destruction of labyrinth, C.
   procedure, C.
Cawthorne-Day labyrinthectomy
CB (cervicobuccal or chronic bronchitis)
CCA (chimpanzee coryza agent)
cecum
   cupular c. of cochlear duct
   cupular ductus cochlearis, c.
   vestibular c. of cochlear duct
   vestibulare ductus cochlearis, c.
cefixime
Ceka
   attachment, C.
   stud, C.
Celestin
   dilator bougie, C.
   esophageal tube, C.
cell
   acoustic hair c.
   agger nasi c.
   auditory c's
   beaker c.
   bristle c's
   chalice c.
   Clara c's
   Claudius c's
   Corti, c's of

cell *(continued)*
   cover c.
   dentin c.
   enamel c.
   encasing c.
   ethmoidal c.
   goblet c.
   gustatory c.
   Hensen c's
   Hurthle c's
   incasing c's
   interdental c's
   interfollicular c's
   lacrimoethmoid c's
   mastoid c.
   Mikulicz c's
   mouth c's
   olfactory c.
   palatine c's
   reserve c's
   Schultze c's
   supporting c's
   taste c's
   Warthin-Finkeldey c's
cell bank
cell button
cell culture
cellophane rales
cellula (pl. cellulae)
cellulae (pl. of cellula)
   ethmoidales osseae, c.
   mastoideae, c.
   pneumaticae tubae auditivae, c.
   pneumaticae tubariae, c.
   tympanicae, c.
cellulitis
celluloid crown
cement
   calcium hydroxide c.
   dental c.
   glass ionomer c.
   organ, c.
   polycarboxylate c.
   resin c.
   root canal c.
   silicate c.

cement *(continued)*
   silicophosphate c.
   zinc oxide-eugenol c.
   zinc phosphate c.
cement base
cement cell
cemental
   caries, c.
   gingiva, c.
cementation
cementicle
   adherent c.
   attached c.
   free c.
   interstitial c.
cementification
cementifying
   fibroma, c.
cementitis
cementoalveolar
cementoblast
cementoblastoma
cementoclasia
cementoclast
cementocyte
cementodentinal
cementoenamel
cementogenesis
cementoid
cementoma
cementopathia
cementoperiostitis
cementosis
cementum
   acellular c.
   afibrillar c.
   cellular c.
   uncalcified c.
central
   aphasia, c.
   caries, c.
   deafness, c.
centric
   bruxism, c.
   jaw relation, c.
   occlusion, c.

centric *(continued)*
   stop, c.
centrolingual
cephalic angle
cephalalgia
   histamine c.
   pharyngotympanic c.
   quadrantal c.
cephalalgic
cephalgia
cephalgic
cephalodynia
cephalogram
cephalogyric
cephalometric angle
cephalometry
cephalopharyngeus
cephaloplegia
cephalostat
cephaloxerogram
cephaloxerography
ceramics
   dental c.
ceramodontia
ceramodontics
ceratohyal
ceratopharyngeal
ceratopharyngeus
cerebellar tonsil
cerebellopontine
cerebral deafness
cerebriform tongue
cerebrospinal
   fluid, c. (CSF)
   rhinorrhea, c.
cerumen
   impacted c.
   inspissated c.
Cerumenex
ceruminal
ceruminolysis
ceruminolytic
   agent, c.
ceruminoma
ceruminosis
ceruminous

ceruminous *(continued)*
   deafness, c.
cervical
   adenitis, c.
   adenopathy, c.
   anchorage, c.
   chain, c.
   esophagus, c.
   lymph nodes, c.
   lymphadenopathy, c.
   spine, c.
   traction, c.
cervices (pl. of cervix)
cervicobregmatic diameter
cervicobuccal (CB)
cervicofacial
   facelift, c.
cervicolabial (CL)
cervicolingual (CL)
cervico-occipital
cervicoplasty
cervix (pl. cervices)
   dentis, c.
   mallei, c.
Cetacaine
Ceylon sore mouth
chain
   cervical c.
   lymphatic c.
   ossicular c.
chaise lounge position
chalazion
chalice cells
chalinoplasty
chamber
   acoustic c.
   dental c.
   pulp c.
   relief c.
chancre
chancroid
chancrous
chapped
Charcot triad
Charcot-Leyden crystals
Charlin syndrome

chasma
Chausse
   III projection, C.
   view, C.
check bite
cheek
   bone, c.
   flap, c.
   retractor, c.
   tooth, c.
cheek-biting
cheekbone
cheesy
   abscess, c.
   bronchitis, c.
Cheever tonsillectomy
cheilectomy
cheilectropion
cheilitis
   actinica, c.
   angular c.
   apostematous c.
   commissural c.
   exfoliativa, c.
   glandularis, c.
   granulomatosa, c.
   impetiginous c.
   migrating c.
   solar c.
   venenata, c.
cheiloangioscopy
cheilocarcinoma
cheilognathopalatoschisis
cheilognathoprosoposchisis
cheilognathoschisis
cheilognathouranoschisis
cheilophagia
cheiloplasty
cheilorrhaphy
cheiloschisis
cheilosis
cheilostomatoplasty
cheilotomy
chemabrasion
chemexfoliation
Chemetron HR-1 Humidity Center

chemical peel
chemodectoma
chemosensory
chemosurgical
chemosurgery
Cherney thyroid nodule
Chernov trcheostomy hook
cherry laurel
cherubism
chessboard graft
Chevalier Jackson
    bougie, C.
    bronchoscope, C.
    esophagoscope, C.
    laryngoscope, C.
    operation, C.
    partial laryngectomy, C.
    speculum, C.
    tracheal tube, C.
chewed
chewing
    force, c.
chew-in record
Cheyne nystagmus
Cheyne-Stokes
    asthma, C.
    nystagmus, C.
chi angle
chicle ulcer
chiclero ulcer
chief cell adenoma
Chievitz organ
child esophagoscope
Child Adult Mist (CAM) Tent
chilitis
chilotomy
chimpanzee coryza agent (CCA)
chin
    cleft c.
    galoche c.
chin augmentation
chin block
chin implant
chin jerk
chin prosthesis
chin protuberance

chin reflex
chin strap
chincap
chip
    graft, c.
    syringe, c.
chipped tooth
chisel
    periodontal c.
chisel scaler
chiseled
Chismani attachment
chloracne
chloroform
chloropercha method
choana (pl. choanae)
choanae (pl. of choana)
    osseae, c.
choanal
    atresia, c.
    polyp, c.
choanoid
choke
    -saver, c.
chokes
choking
cholesteatoma
    tympani, c.
cholesteatomatous
chondrodermatitis
chondroectodermal dysplasia
chondroglossus
chondroma
chondroseptum
Chopart cheiloplasty
chorda (pl. chordae)
    saliva, c.
    tympani, c.
    vocalis, c.
chordae (pl. of chorda)
chordectomy
chorditis
    cantorum, c.
    fibrinosa, c.
    nodosa, c.
    tuberosa, c.

chorditis *(continued)*
    vocalis, c.
choreic tongue
Christ-Siemens-Touraine syndrome
chromatic audition
chromatophore
chromic acid bead
chromorhinorrhea
chronic
    cold, c.
    cough, c.
chronicity
CHT (closed head trauma)
chthonophagia
Chubb tonsil forceps
church-spire projection
Chvostek sign
Chvostek-Weiss sign
Ciaccio glands
cicatricial
cicatrix
    manometric c.
Cicherelli forceps
cigarette
    allergy, c.
    cough, c.
    smoke allergy, c.
Cikloid dressing
cilia
    olfactory c.
ciliary
cinchona
cinchonism
cinebronchography
cine-esophagram
Cinelli nasal osteotome
cionectomy
cionitis
cionoptosis
cionorrhaphy
cionotome
cionotomy
circummandibular
circumoral
    cyanosis, c.
    pallor, c.

circumorbital
circumpulpar dentin
circumtonsillar abscess
cistern
cisterna (pl. cisternae)
cisternae (pl. of cisterna)
cisternography
Citelli syndrome
Citelli-Meltzer punch
Civinini
    canal, C.
    process, C.
C&L intracoronal attachment
CL (cervicolingual)
CLA (cervicolabial)
Cladosporium
Clagett Barrett esophagogastrostomy
clamp
    cotton roll rubber dam c.
    gingival c.
    Joseph c.
    rubber-dam c.
clamp band
clamping habit
Clapton line
Clara cells
Clark classification
clasp
    Adams c.
    arrow c.
    arrowhead c.
    bar c.
    circumferential c.
    continuous c.
    continuous lingual c.
    Crozat c.
clasp arm
    denture, c.
clasp guideline
classification
    Angle c.
    Breslow c.
    Clark c.
    Jewett c.
    Kennedy c.
    Lennert c.

classification *(continued)*
    Lukes-Collins c.
    Rappaport c.
    Skinner c.
Claudius cells
claustra (pl. of claustrum)
claustrum (pl. claustra)
    gutturis, c.
    oris, c.
clausura
cleansing breath
cleft
    alveolar c.
    branchial c.
    craniofacial c.
    facial c.
    gingival c.
    hyobranchial c.
    hyoid c.
    hyomandibular c.
    interdental c.
    nasal c.
    palatal c.
    Stillman c.
    uvular c.
cleft cheek
cleft face
cleft jaw
cleft lip
cleft lip/nose
cleft nose
cleft palate
cleft tongue
cleft uvula
clefting
cleidocranial
    dysostosis, c.
clenching
    habit, c.
    jaw, c. of
    teeth, c. of
Clerf
    laryngeal saw, C.
    laryngoscope, C.
clergyman's sore throat
click stimuli

clicking
    teeth, c.
    tinnitus, c.
clinical crown
clinoid
    process, c.
clipping of frenum linguae
clivogram
clivography
clivus
Cloquet ganglion
close bite
closed
    bite, c.
    head trauma, c. (CHT)
clot
Clot-Stop drain
clotting
    factor, c.
    time, c.
clouding of sinuses
Clouston syndrome
clove oil
coagulate
coagulation
    factor, c.
    time, c.
coagulopathy
Coakley
    antrum curette, C.
    cannula, C.
    curette, C.
    forceps, C.
    frontal sinus cannula, C.
    hemostat, C.
    nasal probe, C.
    probe, C.
    sinus operation, C.
    speculum, C.
    sutures, C.
    trocar, C.
Coakley-Allis forceps
coalescent mastoiditis
coarse breath sounds
coated tongue
cobblestone

cobblestone *(continued)*
    scarring, c.
    tongue, c.
Cobelli glands
cocaine
    pledgets, c.
cocainism
cocainization
cocainized
cochlea (pl. cochleae)
    aqueduct of c.
    cupula of c.
    lamina spiralis ossea, c.
    membranous c.
    modiolus of c.
    scalae of c.
    spiral canal of c.
cochleae (pl. of choclea)
cochlear
    area, c.
    canal, c.
    duct, c.
    electrical stimulation, c.
    eminence, c.
    hydrops, c.
    implant, c.
    joint, c.
    labyrinth, c.
    nerve, c.
    otosclerosis, c.
    potential, c.
    recess of vestibule, c.
    root, c.
    spiral canal, s.
    window, s.
cochleariform
    process, c.
cochleitis
cochleo-orbicular
cochleopalpebral
cochleopupillary
cochleostapedial
cochleotopic
cochleovestibular
cochlitis
codeine

Cody tack perforation of footplate
Coe-pak
Cogan syndrome
cog-tooth of malleus
cogwheel breathing
Cohen nasal-dressing forceps
cohesive gold foil
coil spring
coiled cochlea
cold
    allergic c.
    common c.
    June c.
    rose c.
cold blister
cold-burnished
cold-curing resin
cold mist humidifier
cold pressor test
coldsore
Cole pediatric tube
colla (pl. of collum)
collagen
collar
    bone, c.
    brace, c.
    crown, c.
    incision, c.
collar-button
    abscess, c.
    hook, c.
    tube, c.
Collet syndrome
Collet-Sicard syndrome
colliculi (pl. of colliculus)
colliculicus (pl. colliculi)
Collin tongue forceps
Collins-Mayo mastoid retractor
Collis
    antireflux operation, C.
    mouth gag, C.
collodion
    dressing, c.
colloid goiter
collum (pl. colla)
    dentis, c.

collum (pl. colla) *(continued)*
   mallei, c.
   mandibulae, c.
collunarium
collutory
   Miller c.
coloboma
color
   gustation, c.
   hearing, c.
   taste, c.
colored audition
columella (pl. columellae)
   cochlea, c.
   nasi, c.
columella clamp
columellae (pl. of columella)
columellar type II tympanoplasty
columna
   nasi, c.
columnar-lined esophagus
Colver
   knife, C.
   tonsil forceps, C.
   tonsil hemostat, C.
   tonsil-seizing forceps, C.
Colver-Coakley tonsil forceps
combined aphasia
Commando
   glossectomy, C.
   procedure, C.
commissura (pl. commissurae)
commissurae (pl. of commissura)
commissural
   aphasia, c.
   cheilitis, c.
commissure
   Gudden, c. of
   laryngeal c.
commissurorrhaphy
common
   cold, c.
   cold virus, c.
   dental germ, c.
communicable
Communitrach tube

compaction
compensated
compensating curve
compensatory hypertrophy
compliance
composite
   bonding, c.
   resection, c.
   resin, c.
compound
   anchorage, c.
   flap, c.
   lined flap, c.
compression
   cough, c.
   laryngostenosis, c.
compressor
concave
   facial type, c.
concavity
concavoconcave
concavoconvex
Concept bipolar coagulator
concha (pl. conchae)
   auricle, c. of
   auriculae, c.
   bullosa, c.
   ethmoidal c.
   inferior nasal c.
   inferior turbinate c.
   nasal c.
   nasalis inferior ossea, c.
   nasalis media ossea, c.
   nasalis superior ossea, c.
   nasalis suprema ossea, c.
   nasoturbinal c.
   sphenoidal c.
   sphenoidalis, c.
   superior nasal c.
conchae (pl. of concha)
conchal
   cartilage, c.
   crest, c.
   flap, c.
   mastoid angle, c.
conchectomy

conchiform
conchitis
conchoidal
conchoscope
conchoscopy
conchotome
conchotomy
concrescence
concrete
condensation
condenser
    automatic c.
    gold c.
    mechanical c.
condensing osteitis
conditioning denture
conduction
    aerotympanal c.
    air c.
    air-bone c.
    bone c.
    cranial c.
    osteotympanic c.
    tissue c.
conduction aphasia
conduction deafness
conductive
    deafness, c.
    hearing loss, c.
conductivity
condylar
    axis, c.
    canal, c.
    dystopia, c.
    sag, c.
    shave, c.
condyle
    chord, c.
    mandible, c. of
condylectomy
condyloid
    canal, c.
    process, c.
    tubercle, c.
cone
    elastic c. of larynx

cone *(continued)*
    gutta-percha c.
    long c.
    short c.
confluence
    sinuses, c. of.
confluens
    sinuum, c.
confluent
congestion
    bronchial c.
    nasal c.
congestive
conical tooth
conjunctiva (pl. conjunctivae)
conjunctivae (pl. of conjunctiva)
conjunctivitis
conjunctivocystorhinostomy
connate tooth
connector
    major c.
    minor c.
    saddle c.
connector bar
constrictor
    muscle of pharynx, c.
    pharyngis muscle, c.
contact
    balancing c.
    complete c.
    deflective c.
    initial c.
    occlusal c.
    premature c.
    proximal c.
    proximate c.
    weak c.
    working c.
contact stomatitis
contact surface
continuous
    bar retainer, c.
    lingual clasp, c.
    loop wiring, c.
contour
    gingival c.

contour *(continued)*
    gingival denture c.
contouring
    occlusal c.
contractile ring dysphagia
contralateral
Contralateral Routine of Signals (CROS)
contrast laryngography
contrecoup
control fistula
controlled coughing
contrude
contrusion
conus
    elasticus laryngis, c.
convalescent titer
convergence nystagmus
convergence-retraction nystagmus
Converse
    alar elevator, C.
    bistoury, C.
    chisel, C.
    nasal chisel, C.
    nasal saw, C.
    nasal tip scissors, C.
    otoplasty, C.
    rongeur, C.
    speculum, C.
    tip technique, C.
convex
convexity
convexobasia
convexoconcave
convexoconvex
conveyance
convulsive tic
Cook County tracheal suction tube
cool mist
Cooper nasal ganglia guide
cope
Cope bronchography
coping
copper line
copolymer resin
coralline hydroxyapatite
cord

cord *(continued)*
    dental c.
    enamel c.
    psalterial c.
    vocal c.
cordal
cordectomy
Cordes-New
    elevator, C.
    laryngeal punch, C.
cordopexy
cordotomy
core
    cast c.
corkscrew esophagus
corneomandibular
corneomental
corneopterygoid
corner tooth
corniculate cartilage
cornu (pl. cornua)
    ethmoid c.
    majus ossis hyoidei, c.
    minus ossis hyoidei, c.
cornua (pl. of cornu)
cornual
cornuate
cornucommissural
corona (pl. coronae)
    dental c.
    dentis, c.
coronae (pl. of corona)
coronal
    bleaching, c.
coronale
coronalis
corone
coronion
coronoid
    process, c.
coronoidectomy
coronoidotomy
corpora (pl. of corpus)
corpus (pl. corpora)
    adiposum buccae, c.
    mandibulae, c.

corpus (pl. corpora) *(continued)*
   maxillae, c.
   ossis hyoidei, c.
   ossis sphenoidalis, c.
Corrigan line
corrosive
   esophagitis, c.
   stomatitis, c.
corset platysmaplasty
Corti
   arches, C.
   canal, C.
   ganglion, C.
   membrane, C.
   organ, C.
   rods, C.
   tunnel, C.
cortical
   aphasia, c.
   deafness, c.
   labyrinth, c.
   osteotomy, c.
corticosteroids
corticotomy
corundum
Corwin
   hemostat, C.
   tonsillar forceps, C.
coryza
   allergic c.
   foetida, c.
   oedematosa, c.
coryzavirus
Coschwitz duct
cosmesis
cosmetic
   appearance, c.
   effect, c.
   reconstruction, c.
   surgery, c.
C-osteotomy
Costen syndrome
Cottle
   alar retractor, C.
   clamp, C.
   elevator, C.

Cottle *(continued)*
   forceps, C.
   knife, C.
   nasal-biting rongeur, C.
   osteotome, C.
   pillar retractor, C.
   rasp, C.
   retractor, C.
   saw, C.
   scissors, C.
   soft palate retractor, C.
   speculum, C.
   tenaculum, C.
   Universal nasal saw, C.
Cottle-Arruga forceps
Cottle-Jansen forceps
Cottle-Kazanjian forceps
Cottle-MacKenty septal elevator
Cottle-Nievert retractor
Cottle-Walsham septal straightener
cotton
   -dust asthma, c.
   ear applicator, c.
   nasal applicator, c.
   pellet, c.
   pledget, c.
   roll
   -roll gingivitis, c.
   -roll rubber dam clamp, c.
   swab, c.
   -tipped applicator, c.
   wick, c.
Cotton cartilage graft to cricolaryngeal area
Cotunnius
   aqueduct of C.
   canal of C.
   space of C.
couch grass
cough
   aneurysmal c.
   asthmatic c.
   Balme c.
   barking c.
   brassy c.
   bronchial c.

cough (continued)
   cigarette c.
   compression c.
   croupy c.
   diphtherial c.
   dog c.
   dry c.
   ear c.
   effective c.
   extrapulmonary c.
   hacking c.
   harsh c.
   mechanical c.
   moist c.
   Morton c.
   nonproductive c.
   paroxysmal c.
   privet c.
   productive c.
   pulmonary c.
   reflex c.
   rhonchorous c.
   smoker's c.
   staccato c.
   stomach c.
   Sydenham c.
   tea taster's c.
   trigeminal c.
   uterine c.
   wet c.
   whooping c.
   winter c.
cough drop
cough fracture
cough impulse
cough plate
cough reflex
cough resonance
cough suppressant
cough syncope
cough syrup
coughing
   jag, c.
   spell, c.
coup de sabre
Coupland nasal suction tube
cover
   cells, c.
   dentin, c.
cover with antibiotics
cow face
COWS (cold to the opposite, warm to the same)
coxsackievirus
Co-Xan syrup
cracker test
crackles
crackling
   breath sounds, c.
   jaw, c.
   rales, c.
Craig tonsil-seizing forceps
cranial
   bone, c.
   conduction, c.
cranioaural
craniobuccal
craniocarpotarsal dysplasia
craniodiaphyseal dysplasia
cranioectodermal dysplasia
craniofacial
   angle, c.
   appliance, c.
   axis, c.
   cleft, c.
   disjunction fracture, c.
   dystocia, c.
   dysostosis, c.
   fracture appliance, c.
   microsomia, c.
   suspension wiring, c.
craniognomy
craniograph
craniography
craniomaxillofacial
craniometaphyseal dysplasia
craniometric
craniometry
craniopathy
craniopharyngeal
   canal, c.
   duct, c.

craniopharyngeal *(continued)*
    duct tumor, c.
craniopharyngeus
craniopharyngioma
craniophore
cranioplast
cranioplasty
craniopuncture
craniorachischisis
cranioschisis
cranioscopy
craniosinus
craniosynostosis
craniotelencephalic dysplasia
craniotelencephaly
craniotonoscopy
craniotympanic
cranium
    bifidum, c.
    bifidum occultum, c.
crater
crateriform
craterization
crazing
crease
    ear lobe c.
    nasolabial c.
creola bodies
creosote carbonate
crepitance
crepitant
crepitations (pl. of creps)
creps (pl. crepitations)
crescent
    Giannuzzi, c. of
    sublingual c.
crescentic
crest
    acoustic c.
    acousticofacial c.
    alveolar c.
    arcuate c. of arytenoid cartilage
    basilar c.
    buccinator c.
    cochlear window, c. of
    conchal c.

crest *(continued)*
    dental c.
    ethmoid c.
    ethmoidal c.
    gingival c.
    glandular c. of larynx
    incisor c.
    malar c.
    maxillary c.
    mental c.
    nasal c.
    orbital c.
    palatine c.
    sphenoidal c.
    spiral c. of cochlea
    supramastoid c.
    turbinal c. of palatine bone
    vestibular c.
    zygomatic c.
CREST (calcinosis, Raynaud's phenomenon, esophageal dysmotility, sclerodactyly and telangiectasia)
crevice
    gingival c.
crevicular
cri du chat
crib
    Jackson c.
cribbing
cribra (pl. of cribrum)
cribriform
    plate of ethmoid, c.
cribrum (pl. cribra)
crick
cricoarytenoid
    joint ankylosis, c.
cricoarytenoideus
cricoclavicular line
cricoesophageal
cricoid
    cartilage, c.
    ring, c.
cricoidectomy
cricoidynia
cricopharyngeal
    achalasia syndrome, c.

cricopharyngeus
cricothyreotomy
cricothyroid
    needle puncture, c.
    trocar, c.
cricothyroidotomy
cricothyrotomy
    cannula, c.
    trocar, c.
cricotomy
cricotracheal
cricotracheotomy
Crikelair otoplasty
Crile
    cleft palate clamp, C.
    method, C.
    thyroid double-ended retractor, C.
crisis
    anaphylactic c.
    anaphylactoid c.
    bronchial c.
    laryngeal c.
    pharyngeal c.
    thyroid c.
crista (pl. cristae)
    ampullaris, c.
    arcuata, c.
    conchalis maxillae, c.
    conchalis ossis palatini, c.
    ethmoidalis maxillae, c.
    ethmoidalis ossis palatini, c.
    fenestrae cochleae, c.
    frontalis, c.
    galli, c.
    lacrimalis posterior, c.
    nasalis maxillae, c.
    palatina, c.
    sphenoidalis, c.
    spiralis, c.
    spiralis cochleae, c.
    supramastoidea, c.
    tympanica c.
    vestibuli, c.
cristae (pl. of crista)
cristal
crocodile tongue

Crombie tongue
cromolyn sodium
Cronin
    cleft palate elevator, C.
    palate knife, C.
    procedure, C.
CROS (Contralateral Routine of Signals)
    hearing aid prosthesis
Cross syndrome
Cross-McKusick-Breen syndrome
cross bar elevator
crossbite
    anterior c.
    lingual c.
    posterior c.
    scissors-bite c.
    telescoping c.
crossbite teeth
cross hearing
cross-pin teeth
crossed reflex
croton oil
Crotti thyroid retractor
croup
    catarrhal c.
    diphtheritic c.
    false c.
    membranous c.
    pseudomembranous c.
    spasmodic c.
croup-associated (CA)
    virus, c.
Croupette Child Tent
croup tent
croupous
    bronchitis, c.
    inflammation, c.
    laryngitis, c.
    pharyngitis, c.
    pneumonia, c.
croupy
    cough, c.
Crouzon
    craniofacial dysplasia, C.
    disease, C.
Crowe-Davis mouth gag

crowing breath sounds
crown
  anatomical c.
  artificial c.
  basket c.
  bell c.
  Bonwill c.
  cap c.
  celluloid c.
  clinical c.
  collar c.
  complete c.
  dental c.
  dowel c.
  extra-alveolar c.
  full veneer c.
  gold c.
  half-cap c.
  jacket c.
  open-face c.
  overlay c.
  partial veneer c.
  physiological c.
  pinledge c.
  porcelain c.
  Richmond c.
  shell c.
  tapered c.
  three-quarter c.
  veneer c.
  veneered c.
  window c.
crown drill
crown flask
crownwork
crozat
Crozat
  appliance, C.
  clasp, C.
crura (pl. of crus)
  anterior c. of stapes
  anterius stapedis, c.
  anthelicis, c.
  anthelix, c. of
  breve incudis, c.
  helicus, c.

crura (pl. of crus) *(continued)*
  helix, c. of
  laterale cartilaginis alaris majoris, c.
  long c. of incus
  longus incudis, c.
  mediale, c.
  membranacea, c.
  membranaceum, c.
  ossea, c.
  osseous c.
  osseum commune, c.
  osseum simplex, c.
  posterior c. of stapes
  posterius stapedis, c.
  short c. of incus
  simple membranous c. of semicircular duct
crural
  canal of Henle, c.
cruroplasty
crus (pl. crura)
Cryer elevator
cryocautery
cryostat
cryosurgery
cryosurgical
cryotherapy
crypt
  bony c.
  dental c.
  enamel c.
  palatine tonsil, c's of
  pharyngeal tonsil, c's of
  tongue, c's of
  tonsillar c.
  tooth cc.
crypta (pl. cryptae)
cryptae (pl. of crypta)
cryptic tonsils
cryptotia
crystal
  apatite c.
  asthma c's
  Charcot-Leyden c's
  ear c.
CSF (cerebrospinal fluid)

C-shaped deflection
cuajani
cued speech
cuff tracheostomy
cuffed
    endotracheal tube, c.
    tracheostomy tube, c.
Cukier nasal forceps
Cullom septal forceps
Cullom-Mueller adenotome
cuneiform
    cartilage, c.
    tubercle, c.
cup ear
cup-shaped ear forceps
cupid's bow
cupola
cupula (pl. cupulae)
    cochlea, c. of
    cochleae, c.
    cristae ampullaris, c.
cupulae (pl. of cupula)
cupular
    space, c.
cupulogram
cupulolithiasis
cupulometry
curled enamel
curling
currant jelly sputum
curettage
    apical c.
    gingival c.
    periapical c.
    subgingival c.
    surgical c.
    ultrasonic c.
Curschmann spirals
curve
    alignment c.
    anti-Monson c.
    audibility c.
    buccal c.
    compensating c.
    dental c.
    labial c.

curve *(continued)*
    Monson c.
    occlusion, c. of
    reverse c.
    Spee, c. of
curvilinear
Cushing
    forceps, C.
    staphylorrhaphy elevator, C.
    syndrome, C.
cushingoid facies
cushion
cusp
    Carabelli c.
    dental c.
cusp angle
cusp height
cusp plane
cuspal
cuspid
    deciduous c.
    mandibular c.
    maxillary c.
cuspid tooth
cuspidate
cuspides (pl. of cuspis)
cuspidor
cuspis (pl. cuspides)
    dentalis, c.
cuspless tooth
cutaneous asthma
cuticle
    acquired c.
    attachment c.
    dental c.
    enamel c.
    secondary c.
cuticula
    dentis, c.
Cutler-Beard bridge flap
cutting
    Bovie knife, c.
    current, c.
    disk, c.
    edge, c.
    teeth, c.

cuttlefish disk
cyano-acrylate
cyanosed
cyanosis
   central c.
   circumoral c.
cyanotic
Cyklokapron
cylindroma
cymba (pl. cymbae)
   conchae auriculae, c.
cymbae (pl. of cymba)
cymbiform
cynanche
   maligna, c.
   tonsillaris, c.
cynic spasm
cyst
   alveolar c.
   apical c.
   branchial c.
   branchiogenous c.
   cervical c.
   congenital c.
   craniobuccal c.
   craniopharyngeal c.
   dental c.
   dentigerous c.
   dermoid c.
   eruption c.

cyst *(continued)*
   gingival c.
   globulomaxillary c.
   incisive canal c.
   lateral periodontal c.
   median anterior maxillary c.
   median mandibular c.
   median palatal c.
   nasoalveolar c.
   nasolabial c.
   nasopalatine duct c.
   odontogenic c.
   periapical c.
   periodontal c.
   preauricular c.
   primordial c.
   radicular c.
   residual c.
   sublingual c.
   suprasellar c.
   thyroglossal c.
   thyrolingual c.
   Tornwaldt c.
cystic
   fibrosis, c.
   hygroma, c.
cytisism
cytomegalovirus
Czermak spaces

Additional entries

D

dacryoadenectomy
dacryoadenotomy
dacryoblennorrhea
dacryocystitis
dacryocystitome
dacryocystoblennorrhea
dacryocystocele
dacryocystography
dacryocystoptosis
dacryocystorhinostenosis
dacryocystorhinostomy
    needle, d.
    retractor, d.
    trephine, d.
dacryocystorhinotomy
dacryocystosyringotomy
dacryocystotome
dacryocystotomy
dacryolith
dacryolite
dacryolithiasis
dacryon
dacryorhinocystotomy
dacryorhinocystotomy
dacryosinusitis
dacryosolenitis
dacryostenosis
dacryosyrinx
dactylocostal rhinoplasty
DAG (distoaxiogingival)
DAI (distoaxioincisal)
Dalbo
    attachment, D.
    stud, D.
dam
dander
Daniels tonsillectome
Dann-Jennings mouth gag
DAO (distoaxio-occlusal)
Darwin ear
darwinian
    apex, d.
    ear, d.

darwinian *(continued)*
    tubercle, d.
D'Assumpcao rhytidoplasty marker
Daubenton angle
Dautrey sagittal split osteotomy
Davis
    bronchoscope, D.
    mouth gag, D.
    tonsillar hemostat, D.
    tonsillar knife, D.
    tonsillar needle, D.
    tooth plate, D.
Davis-Crowe mouth gag
Davis and Kitlowski otoplasty
Day
    attic cannula, D.
    ear hook, D.
    electrocoagulation, D.
    operation, D.
    tonsillar knife, D.
dB (decibel)
DB (distobuccal)
DBO (distobucco-occlusal)
DBP (distobuccopulpal)
DC (distocervical)
deaf
    -mute, d.
    -mutism, d.
    point, d.
deafness
    acoustic trauma d.
    Alexander d.
    apoplectiform d.
    aviator's d.
    bass d.
    boilermaker's d.
    central d.
    cerebral d.
    ceruminous d.
    conduction d.
    congenital d.
    cortical d.
    functional d.

deafness *(continued)*
  genetic d.
  high frequency d.
  hysterical d.
  inner ear d.
  labyrinthine d.
  malarial d.
  Michel d.
  midbrain d.
  middle ear d.
  mixed d.
  Mondini d.
  music d.
  nerve d.
  neural d.
  occupational d.
  organic d.
  ototoxic d.
  pagetoid d.
  paradoxic d.
  perceptive d.
  postlingual d.
  prelingual d.
  psychic d.
  Scheibe d.
  sensorineural d.
  tone d.
  toxic d.
  transmission d.
  traumatic d.
  vascular d.
  word d.
deafness-onychodystrophy-osteodystrophy retardation (DOOR) syndrome
deallergization
Dean
  applicator, D.
  ear snare, D.
  hemostat, D.
  knife, d.
  mastoid rongeur, D.
  periosteotome, D.
  tonsillar forceps, D.
Dean-Shallcross tonsil-seizing forceps
debanding
Debove membrane

debride
debridement
  canal d.
  epithelial d.
  root canal d.
debris
decalcification
decalcify
decay
  tone d.
  tooth d.
decayed
decibel (dB)
deciduous
  cuspid, d.
  teeth, d.
Decker
  microsurgery forceps, D.
  pituitary rongeur, D.
decongestant
decongestive
DeCourcy goiter clamp
decussate
decussatio (pl. decussationes)
decussation
decussationes (pl. of decussatio)
dedentition
Dedo laryngoscope
Dedo-Jako microlaryngoscope
Dedo-Pilling laryngoscope
de-epithelialization
de-epithelialize
DEF (decayed, extracted and filled)
  index, D.
  teeth, D.
deflective contact
defluxion
degloved
degloving
deglutible
deglutition
  apnea, d.
  mechanism, d.
  murmur, d.
deglutitive
deglutitory

degustation
dehiscence
    root d.
dehumidifier
dehumidify
Deiter nucleus
Dejerine syndrome
Delaborde tracheal dilator
deLange syndrome
delayed
    dentition, d.
    flap, d.
DeLee
    tracheal catheter, D.
    tracheal trap, D.
    trap meconium aspirator, D.
DeLee'd
Delphian node
demarcate
demarcating clamp
demarcation
Demarquay sign
Demel and Ruttin otoplasty
demineralization
deMorsier syndrome
deMorsier-Gauthier syndrome
demutization
denasality
Dench
    ear, D.
    ear curette, D.
    nebulizer, D.
dendritic
Denhardt mouth gag
Denhardt-Dingman mouth gag
Denholz appliance
Denker procedure
Dennis bipolar cautery
Denonvillier operation
Denonvillier-Joseph procedure
dens (pl. dentes)
    axis, d.
    bicuspidis, d.
    caninus, d.
    deciduus, d.
    epistrophei, d.

dens (pl. dentes) *(continued)*
    incisivus, d.
    in dente, d.
    invaginatus, d.
    molaris, d.
    permanens, d.
    premolaris, d.
    sapientiae, d.
    serotinus, d.
dentagra
dental
    abscess, d.
    adhesive, d.
    adnexa, d.
    alveolus, d.
    amalgam, d.
    anesthesia, d.
    ankylosis, d.
    appliance, d.
    arch, d.
    arch bar, d.
    arch bar frame, d.
    artery, d.
    assistant, d.
    bridge, d.
    bur, d.
    calculus, d.
    canaliculi, d.
    canals, d.
    caries, d.
    cast, d.
    cavity, d.
    cement, d.
    chart, d.
    consonant, d.
    cord, d.
    corona, d.
    crest, d.
    crown, d.
    crypt, d.
    curve, d.
    cuticle, d.
    debridement, d.
    disclosing agent, d.
    disk, d.
    drill, d.

dental *(continued)*
   dysfunction, d.
   elevator, d.
   enamel, d.
   engine, d.
   engineering, d.
   excavator, d.
   exostosis, d.
   explorator, d.
   extirpation, d.
   extraction, d.
   filling, d.
   fistula, d.
   flange, d.
   floss, d.
   fluorosis, d.
   follicular cyst, d.
   forceps, d.
   formula, d.
   furrow, d.
   geriatrics, d.
   germ, d.
   granuloma, d.
   handpiece, d.
   hygiene, d.
   hygienist, d.
   impaction, d.
   implant, d.
   implantology, d.
   impression, d.
   index, d.
   instruments, d.
   interproximal survey, d.
   knife, d.
   lamina, d.
   materials, d.
   molares, d.
   mold, d.
   neck, d.
   nerve, d.
   occlusal, d.
   panoramic, d.
   periapical, d.
   plaque, d.
   plate, d.
   pliers, d.

dental *(continued)*
   prosthesis, d.
   prophylaxis, d.
   pulp, d.
   radiography, d.
   repair, d.
   restoration, d.
   restorative surgery, d.
   ridge, d.
   roll, d.
   root, d.
   root end cyst, d.
   sac, d.
   sealant, d.
   senescence, d.
   shelf, d.
   splint, d.
   syringe, d.
   tape, d.
   tool, d.
   tophus, d.
   trephination, d.
   tubules, d.
   wax, d.
dentalgia
dentaphone
dentary center
dentate
dentes (pl. of dens)
   acustici, d.
   acuti, d.
   canini, d.
   de Chiaie, d.
   decidui, d.
   incisivi, d.
   molares, d.
   permanentes, d.
   premolares, d.
Dentatus ARL
dentia
   praecox, d.
   tarda, d.
dentibuccal
denticle
   adherent d.
   attached d.

denticle *(continued)*
    embedded d.
    false d.
    free d.
    interstitial d.
    true d.
denticulated
dentification
dentiform
dentifrice
dentigerous
    follicular cyst, d.
dentilabial
dentilingual
dentimeter
dentin
    adventitious d.
    calcified d.
    circumpulpar d.
    cover d.
    functional d.
    hereditary opalescent d.
    interglobular d.
    intertubular d.
    irregular
    mantle d.
    opalescent d.
    primary d.
    reparative d.
    sclerotic d.
    secondary d.
    secondary irregular d.
    secondary regular d.
    tertiary d.
    transparent d.
dentin bridge
dentin cells
dentin crystal alteration
dentinal
    canaliculi, d.
    canals, d.
    caries, d.
    cartilage, d.
    fibers, d.
    matrix, d.
    sheath of Neumann, d.

dentinal *(continued)*
    tubules, d.
dentinalgia
dentine
dentinification
dentinitis
dentinoblast
dentinoblastoma
dentinocemental
dentinoclast
dentinoenamel
dentinogenesis
    imperfecta, d.
dentinogenic
dentinogingival
dentinoid
dentinoma
dentinosteoid
dentinum
dentiparous
dentist
dentistry
    cosmetic d.
    esthetic d.
    forensic, d.
    four-handed d.
    geriatric d.
    hospital d.
    legal d.
    operative d.
    pediatric d.
    preventive d.
    prosthetic d.
    prosthodontic d.
    psychosomatic d.
    restorative d.
dentition
    artificial d.
    deciduous d.
    delayed d.
    diphyodont d.
    heterodont d.
    homodont d.
    mixed d.
    monophyodont d.
    natural d.

dentition *(continued)*
   permanent d.
   polyphyodont d.
   precocious d.
   predeciduous d.
   premature d.
   primary d.
   retarded d.
   secondary d.
   transitional d.
dentitional
   odontectomy, d.
dentoalveolar
   abscess, d.
   joint, d.
dentoalveolitis
dentofacial
dentography
dentoid
dentoidin
dentolegal
dentoma
dentomechanical
dentonomy
dentosurgical
dentotropic
dentulous
denture
   clasp d.
   complete d.
   conditioning d.
   fixed partial d.
   full d.
   immediate d.
   immediate-insertion d.
   implant d.
   interim d.
   lower d.
   overlay d.
   partial d.
   permanent d.
   provisional d.
   removable partial d.
   telescopic d.
   temporary d.
   transitional d.

denture *(continued)*
   trial d.
   unilateral partial d.
denture adhesive
denture base
denture base saddle
denture-bearing area
denture brush
denture flask
denture foundation area
denture impression
denture irritation
denture magnet
denture splint
denture stomatitis
denture-supporting area
dentures
denturism
denturist
Denver nasal splint
deoxyribonucleic acid (DNA)
deposit
   calcareous d.
   tooth d.
depressed fracture
depression
   nasal bone d.
depressor
   alae nasi muscle, d.
   anguli oris muscle, d.
   labii inferioris muscle, d.
deQuervain thyroiditis
Derf ear knife
Derlacki
   chisel, D.
   ear curette, D.
   gouge, D.
   knife, D.
   mobilizer, D.
   tympanoplasty, D.
Derlacki-Shambaugh chisel
dermabraded
dermabrader
dermabrasion
dermabrasion
dermatitis

dermatitis *(continued)*
    eczematous d.
    medicamentosis, d.
dermatoautoplasty
dermatoheteroplasty
dermatoplasty
dermatome
dermoid
    tumor, d.
dermoidectomy
dermoplasty
DeRoaldes nasal speculum
DES (diffuse esophageal spasm)
desalivation
DeSalle line
desensitization
desensitize
desiccant
desiccate
desiccation
desiccator
desmodontium
d'Espine sign
desquamation
desquamative gingivitis
dethyroidism
dethyroidize
detrition
detritus
deux lambeaux procedure
deviated
    nasal septum, d.
    nasal tip, d.
    trachea, d.
deviation
    nasoseptal d.
    tongue d.
    tracheal d.
device
    central-bearing d.
    central-bearing tracing d.
deVilbiss nebulizer
devitalization
devitalize
devitalized tissue
deviated

deviated *(continued)*
    nasal septum, d.
deviation
    nasoseptal d.
    tongue d.
    tracheal d.
devorative
dewlap
dexapolyspectran
dextrality
dextraural
dextromethorphan
DG (distogingival)
diameter
    bigonial d.
    biparietal d.
    bitemporal d.
    bizygomatic d.
    buccolingual d.
    cervicobregmatic d.
    frontomental d.
    labiolingual d.
    mentobregmatic d.
    mesiodistal d.
    occipitofrontal d.
    occipitomental d.
diabetic ear
diamond
    bur, d.
    disk, d.
    drill, d.
    fraise, d.
diapason
diastema (pl. diastemata)
diastemata (pl. of diastema)
diastematocrania
diastolization
diathermy
diatoric tooth
diazone
Dibbell cleft lip-nasal revision
dicheilia
die
    amalgam d.
    electroformed d.
    electroplated d.

die *(continued)*
    plated d.
    waxing d.
die plate
Dieffenbach otoplasty
Dieffenbach-Szymanowski-Kuhnt procedure
Dieffenbach-Warren technique
Dieffenbach-Webster sliding cheek procedure
difference limen (DL) test
Diflucan
diffuse esophageal spasm (DES)
digastricus
DiGeorge syndrome
digestive
    apparatus, d.
    tract, d.
diglossia
dignathus
diisocyanate asthma
dilaceration
Dilantin
    gingivitis, D.
    hyperplasia, D.
dilated odontoma
dilatancy
dilatation
    esophageal d.
dilation
dilator
dimenhydrinate
Dimetane
Dimetapp
Dimitry dacryocystorhinostomy trephine
DIMOAD (diabetes insipidus, diabetes mellitus, optic atrophy, and deafness)
Dingman
    elevator, D.
    forceps, D.
    mouth gag, D.
    ostectomy, D.
    osteotome, D.
    retractor, D.
    wire passer, D.

Dingman *(continued)*
    zygoma elevator, D.
    zygoma hook, d.
Dingman-Denhardt mouth gag
dinical
dinitrogen monoxide
Dintenfass ear kinfe
diphenhydramine
diphenylhydantoin gingivitis
diphonia
diphtheria
    laryngeal d.
diphtherial
    cough, d.
    tonsillitis, d.
diphtheric
diphtherin
diphtheritic
    croup, d.
    laryngitis, d.
    pharyngitis, d.
    stomatitis, d.
diphtheroid
diphtherotoxin
diphthong
diphthongia
diphyodont dentition
diplacusis
    binaural d.
    binauralis dysharmonica, d.
    binauralis echoica, d.
    disharmonic d.
    echo d.
    monaural d.
    monauralis, d.
diplegia
    facial d.
    masticatory d.
diploe
diploetic
diplophonia
diplopia
direct
    filling resin, d.
    laryngoscopy, d.
    -vision adenotome, d.

disci (pl. of discus)
disclosing agent
discoid
disconnection syndrome
discrimination
discus (pl. disci)
disequilibrium
dish face
dished
    face, d.
    nose, d.
disharmony
disimpaction
disjunction
disjunctive nystamus
disk
    abrasive d.
    Blake d.
    Carborundum d.
    cutting d.
    cuttlefish d.
    dental d.
    diamond d.
    emery d.
    polishing d.
    sandpaper d.
disocclude
disocclusion
dissector
dissociated nystagmus
distal
    esophageal ring, d.
    esophagectomy, d.
    esophagus, d.
distance
    interarch d.
    interocclusal d.
    interridge d.
distant flap
distoaxiogingival (DAG)
distoaxioincisal (DAI)
distoaxio-occlusal (DAO)
distobuccal (DB)
distobuccopulpal (DBP)
distobucco-occlusal (DBO)
distocervical (DC)
distoclination
distoclusal
distoclusion
distogingival (DG)
distolabial (DLA)
distolabioincisal (DLAI)
distolingual (DL)
distolinguoincisal (DLI)
distolinguo-occlusal (DLO)
distolinguopulpal (DLP)
distomia
distomolar
distomus
disto-occlusal (DO)
disto-occlusion
distoplacement
distopulpal (DP)
distopulpolabial (DPLA)
distopulpolingual (DPL)
distortor
    oris, d.
distoversion
distraction
ditched filling
Dittrich plugs
diverticula (pl. of diverticulum)
diverticulum (pl. diverticula)
    esophageal d.
    Kirchner d.
    laryngeal d.
    Pertik d.
    pharyngoesophageal d.
    Rokitansky d.
    thyroid d.
    tracheal d.
    traction d.
    Zenker d.
diving goiter
Dix-Hallpike test
Dixon
    nasal speculum, D.
    retractor, D.
dizziness
dizzy
DL (difference limen or distolingual)
DLA (distolabial)

DLAI (distolabioincisal)
DLI (distolinguoincisal)
DLO (distolinguo-occlusal)
DLP (distolinguopulpal)
DMF (delayed, missing, and filled)
    index, D.
    teeth, D.
DNA (deoxyribonucleic acid)
    engineering, D.
    histogram, D.
    library, D.
    -ploidy, D.
    plotting, D.
DNCB skin test
DO (disto-occlusal)
Doc's ear plugs
Doerfler Stewart Test
dog cough
dogear
dogleg
Dohlman incus hook
Dolder bar
doll's eye sign
Dommanate
Donaldson
    eustachian tube, D.
    myringotomy tube, D.
    Silastic ear tube, D.
    Teflon tube, D.
Donohue syndrome
donor island harvesting
DOOR (deafness-onychodystrophy-osteodystrophy-retardation) syndrome
Doppler flowmeter
Dorello canal
Dorrance palatal pushback
dorsal
    hump, d.
    root entry zone, d. (DREZ)
    strut, d.
Dorsey tongue depressor
dorsum
    linguae, d.
    nasi, d.
dose-pack
Dott

Dott *(continued)*
    mouth gag, D.
    procedure, D.
Dott-Kilner mouth gag
dotted tongue
double
    chin, d.
    disharmonic hearing, d.
    -door tongue flap, d.
    lip, d.
    pedicle flap, d.
    tongue, d.
    voice, d.
douche
    Bermingham nasal d.
    nasal d.
Douglas
    graft, D.
    knife, d.
    nasal scissors, D.
    tongue suture, D.
dowel
    crown, d.
Down syndrome
downbeat nystagmus
Downs Y axis
doxycycline
Doyen
    mouth gag, D.
    raspatory, D.
Doyen-Jansen mouth gag
DP (distopulpal)
DPL (distopulpolingual)
DPLA (distopulpolabial)
DPT (diphtheria, pertussis, and tetanus)
drag
Dragstedt graft
draining sinus
Dramamine
draw-cut technique
DREZ (dorsal root entry zone)
drift
drifting tooth
drill
drilling
Drinker respirator

drooling
droplet
   infection, d.
dropper
   medicine d.
drops
   ear d.
   nose d.
Dr. Marsh Robinson mandibular procedure
droplet enamel cells
drum
   elevator, d.
   elevator knife, d.
   membrane, d.
   probe, d.
   scraper, d.
drumhead
dry
   bronchitis, d.
   caries, d.
   catarrh, d.
   cough, d.
   heaves, d.
   mouth, d.
   socket, d.
   tongue, d.
DTP (diphtheria, tetanus, and pertussis)
dual distal lighted laryngoscope
Duane syndrome
Dubreuil-Chambardel syndrome
duct
   acoustic d.
   Bartholin d.
   Blasius d.
   branchial d's
   cochlear d.
   Coschwitz d.
   craniopharyngeal d.
   endolymphatic d.
   His, d. of
   incisive d.
   incisor d.
   lacrimal d.
   lacrimonasal d.
   lingual d.

duct *(continued)*
   nasal d.
   nasofrontal d.
   nasolacrimal d.
   nasopharyngeal d.
   parotid d.
   Rivinus, d's. of
   sacculoutricular d.
   semicircular d's
   Steno, d. of
   Stensen d.
   sublingual d's
   submandibular d.
   submaxillary d. of Wharton
   tear d's
   thyroglossal d.
   thyrolingual d.
   utriculosaccular d.
   Vater, d. of
   Walther d's.
   Wharton d.
ductal
ducti (pl. of ductus)
ductus (pl. ducti)
   cochlearis, d.
   endolymphaticus, d.
   incisivus, d.
   lacrimales, d.
   lingualis, d.
   nasolacrimalis, d.
   parotideus, d.
   reuniens, d.
   semicirculares, d.
   sublingualis, d.
   submandibularis, d.
   thyroglossalis, d.
   utricosaccularis d.
Duel-Ballance facial nerve repair
Dufourmental
   forceps, D.
   rongeur, D.
Dulaney antral cannula
dull light reflex
dumb
   rabies, d.
Dumbach Titanium mesh

dumbness
Dumon
   bronchoscope, D.
   trachea tube, D.
Dumon-Harrell
   bronchoscope, D.
   tracheal tube, D.
Dunn tongue depressor
Duplay nasal speculum
Duplay-Lynch nasal speculum
Dupuy-Dutemps blepharoplasty
dural abscess
Durapatite
Durham
   tracheostomy tube, D.
   tracheotomy trocar, C.
duskiness
dusky
dust
   bone d.
   ear d.
dust asthma
dust-borne
dwarfed enamel
dye laser
Dyke-Davidoff syndrome
dynamic facial skin lines
dysacousia
dysacousma
dysacusia
dysacusis
dysallilognathia
dysantigraphia
dysarthria
dysarthric
dysaudia
dyscephaly
dyscrinic rhinitis
dysequilibrium
dysesthesia
   auditory d.
dysfluency
dysgeusia
dysgnathia
dyslalia
dyslexia

dysodontiasis
dysosmia
dysostosis
   acrofacial d.
   cleidocranial d.
   cleidocranialis, d.
   cleidodigitalis, d.
   craniocerebral d.
   craniofacial d.
   craniofacialis hereditaria, d.
   cranio-orbitofacialis d.
   Crouzon craniofacial d.
   mandibularis, d.
   mandibulofacial d.
   Nager acrofacial d.
   orodigitofacial d.
dysphagia
   constricta, d.
   contractile ring d.
   inflammatoria, d.
   lusoria, d.
   nervosa, d.
   paralytica, d.
   sideropenic c.
   spastica, d.
   valsalviana, d.
   vallecular d.
dysphagic
dysphagy
dysphasia
dusphasic
dysphemia
dysphonia
   clericorum, d.
   plicae ventricularis, d.
   puberum, d.
   spasmodic d.
   spastica, d.
dysphrasia
dysplasia
   anhydrotic ectodermal d.
   anteroposterior facial d.
   chondroectodermal d.
   cleidocranial d.
   craniocarpotarsal d.
   craniodiaphyseal d.

dysplasia *(continued)*
- cranioectodermal d.
- craniometaphyseal d.
- craniotelencephalic d.
- Crouzon craniofacial d.
- dental d.
- dentinal d.
- dentoalveolar d.
- ectodermal d.
- encephalo-ophthalmic d.
- faciocardiomelic d.
- fibrous d. of jaw
- frontonasal d.
- hidrotic ectodermal d.
- hypohidrotic ectodermal d.

dysplasia *(continued)*
- linguifacialis, d.
- mandibulosacral d.
- oculoauricular d.
- oculoauriculovertebral d.
- oculodentodigital d.
- oculodentodigitalis, d.
- oculodento-osseous d.
- ophthalmomandibulomelic d.

dysplastic
dyspnea
dyspneic
dysprosody
dystimbria

Additional entries

E

EAC (external auditory canal)
Eagleton extrapetrosal drainage
EAHF (eczema, asthma, hay fever)
EAM (external auditory meatus)
ear
    acute e.
    aviator's e.
    Aztec e.
    bat e.
    Blainville e's
    Cagot e.
    cauliflower e.
    cup e.
    Darwin e.
    diabetic e.
    external e.
    glue e.
    hairy e's
    Hong Kong e.
    hot weather e.
    inner e.
    insane e.
    internal e.
    lop e.
    middle e.
    Morel e.
    Mozart e.
    outer e.
    pierced e.
    prizefighter e.
    satyr e.
    scroll e.
    Singapore e.
    swimmer's e.
    tank e.
    tropical e.
    Wildermuth e.
ear applicator
ear basin
ear bistoury
ear block
ear bone
ear bougie

ear canal
ear cartilage
ear cavity
ear cough
ear crystal
ear cup
ear curette
ear cut snare wire
ear dissector
ear drops
ear dust
ear elevator
ear forceps
ear hook
ear knife
ear loop
ear loupe
ear marker
ear-minded
ear mobilizer
ear oximeter
ear oximetry
ear piercing
ear pinna
ear pinna prosthesis
ear piston
ear piston prosthesis
ear plug
ear probe
ear punch
ear punch forceps
ear reconstruction
ear rongeur
ear scissors
ear scoop
ear setback
ear snare
ear speculum
ear spoon
ear suction tube
ear syringe
ear trumpet
ear tubes

ear wick
earache
eardrops
eardrum
   elevator, e.
   injection of e.
   retraction of e.
   ruptured e.
ear-grasping forceps
earlobe
   crease, e.
   keloid, e.
earring
earthy tongue
earwash
earwax
Eaton
   agent, E.
   nasal speculum, e.
Ebner
   fibrils, E.
   glands, E.
   lines, E.
ebur
   dentis, e.
eburnation
   dentin, e. of
eburneous
eburnitis
eccentric jaw relation
ecchymosis
ecchymotic
echo dyplacusis
ECHO (enteric cytopathogenic human orphan) virus
echoacousia
echolalia
echophony
echophotony
echopraxis
echovirus
Eckstein-Kleinschmidt otoplasty
ecthyma
ectodermal dysplasia
ectopterygoid
ectropion

eczema, asthma, hay fever (EAHF)
edentate
edentia
edentulate
edentulous
Eder esophagoscope
Eder-Hufford esophagoscope
edge
   bevel e.
   chamber e.
   cutting e.
   denture e.
   incisal e.
edge-strength
edgewise appliance
Edinger-Westphal nucleus
Edlich lavage tube
Edwards syndrome
EEC (ectrodactyly-ectodermal dysplasia-clefting) syndrome
EENT (eyes, ears, nose, and throat)
E.E.S. (erythromycin ethylsuccinate)
effective cough
EG (esophagogastric)
   junction, E.
EGD (esophagogastroduodenoscopy)
EGJ (esophagogastric junction)
egobronchophony
egophony
Ehmke
   ear prosthesis, E.
   platinum Teflon prosthesis, E.
Ehrenritter ganglion
Eicken method
eight-lumen esophageal manometry catheter
Eikenella corrodens
Einhorn esophageal dilator
Eitner otoplasty
elastic
   intermaxillary e.
   intramaxillary e.
   vertical e.
elastic band fixation
elastic cartilage
elastic cone of larynx

elastic fibers in sputum
elastomer
elective mutism
electrical nystagmus
electrocochleogram
electrocochleograph
electrocochleographic audiometry
electrocochleograpy
electrodermal audiometry
electrodesiccation
electroformed die
electrofulgurate
electrofulguration
electrogustometry
electromyography
electroneuronogram
electroneuronography
electronystagmogram (ENG)
electronystagmography
electro-oculogram
electro-olfactogram (EOG)
electroplated die
electropneumatotherapy
electroresection
electrosalivogram
electroscission
electrosection
electrostimulation
electrosurgery
   pencil, e.
electrosurgical
   knife, e.
electrotome
elephantiasis
   gingivae, e.
elevator
   angular e.
   apical e.
   cross bar e.
   Cryer e.
   dental e.
   malar e.
   periosteum e.
   root e.
   screw e.
   straight e.

elevator *(continued)*
   T-bar e.
   wedge e.
elinguation
elixir
   terpin hydrate, e. (ETH)
   terpin hydrate with codeine, e. (ETH/C)
Elixophyllin
elongation
Elschnig blepharorrhaphy
Elsner asthma
emalloid
embed
embedded
embrasure
Emerson bronchoscope
emery
   disk, e.
emesis
emetic
emetine
emetism
EMG (exophthalmos-macroglossia-gigantism)
eminence
   arytenoid e.
   canine e.
   cochlear e.
   concha, e. of
   facial e. of eminentia teres
   frontal e.
   hypobranchial e.
   jugular e.
   malar e.
   maxilla, e. of
   nasal e.
   orbital e. of zygomatic bone
   pyramidal e.
   thyroid e.
   triangular e.
   triquetral fossa, e. of
eminenectomy
eminentia (pl. eminentiae)
   articularis ossis temporalis, e.
   conchae, e.

eminentia (pl. eminentiae) *(continued)*
    facialis, e.
    fallopii, e.
    fossae triangularis auriculae, e.
    hypoglossi, e.
    maxillae, e.
    orbitalis ossis zygomatici, e.
    pyramidalis, e.
    scaphae, e.
    teres, e.
    triangularis, e.
eminentiae (pl. of eminentia)
emissaria (pl. of emissarium)
emissarium (pl. emissaria)
    mastoideum, e.
emphysema
emphysematous
    asthma, e.
empiric antibiotics
empyema
empyemic
empyesis
en plaque
enamel
    aprismatic e.
    brown e.
    cervical e.
    curled e.
    dental e.
    dwarfed e.
    gnarled e.
    hereditary brown e.
    hypoplastic e.
    mottled e.
    nanoid e.
    straight e.
enamel builder
enamel cap
enamel caries
enamel cells of teeth
enamel cord
enamel crypt
enamel cuticle
enamel drop
enamel epithelium
enamel germ

enamel hypocalcification
enamel hypoplasia
enamel knot
enamel lamellae
enamel navel
enamel niche
enamel organ
enamel pearl
enamel prism
enameloblast
enameloblastoma
enamelogenesis
    imperfecta, e.
enameloma
enamelum
enanthem
enanthema
en bloc
encasing cell
encephalitis
encephalocele
enchondroma
encrusted tongue
endaural
    approach, e.
    curette, e.
    incision, e.
    retractor, e.
    rongeur, e.
    speculum, e.
endemic goiter
endobronchial
endobronchitis
endodontia
endodontic implant
endodontics
endodontist
endodontitis
endodontium
endodontologist
endodontology
endoesophageal
    prosthesis, e.
endoesophagitis
endognathion
endolabyrinthitis

endolaryngeal
  mold, e.
endolarynx
endolymph
endolympha
endolymphatic
  duct, e.
  hydrops, e.
  labyrinth, e.
endomastoiditis
endonasal
endorhinitis
endoscope
endoscopy
  peroral e.
endosseal
endosseous implant
endosteal
  implant, e.
  implant anchor, e.
endothermy
endothyropexy
endotoscope
endotoscopy
endotracheal (ET)
  cuffed e. tube
  curette, e.
  insufflation, e.
  intubation, e.
  stripper, e.
  tube, e.
endotracheitis
end-position nystagmus
en face
ENG (electronystagmogram)
engine
  dental e.
  high-speed e.
  ultraspeed e.
English rhinoplasty
en masse
enostosis
enostotic
en plaque
ENT (ears, nose, and throat)
  chair, E.

entacoustic
entocone
entomion
entorbital fissure
entotic
  sound, e.
entotympanic
enucleate
enucleation
enucleator
envelope flap
environmental
  allergen, e.
  control, e.
Eoerfler-Stewart test
EOG (electro-olfactogram)
EOM (extraocular muscles)
EOMI (extraocular muscles intact)
eosinophilia
eosinophilic granuloma
epactal cartilage
eparterial
ephedrine
epi (epinephrine)
ephippium
epibulbar
  dermoid, e.
epicanthal
  fold, e.
epicanthic
  fold, e.
epicanthine
epicanthus
epidemic
  hiccup, e.
  stomatitis, e.
epidermoid
epiesophageal
epiglottectomy
epiglottic
epiglottidean
epiglottidectomy
epiglottiditis
epiglottis
epiglottitis
epiglottopexy

76   epignathous

epignathous
epignathus
epihyal
epihyoid
epimandibular
epiotic
   center, e.
epinephrine
epipharyngeal
epipharyngitis
epipharynx
epiphora
Epistat double balloon
epistaxis
   apple-packer's e.
epistaxis balloon
epistaxis tamponade
epithelial
   attachment of Gottlieb, e.
   rest, e.
epithelialization
epithelialize
epithelium
   attachment e.
   Barrett e.
   ductus semicircularis, e.
   enamel e.
   gingival e.
   junctional e.
   laminated e.
   olfactory e.
   reduced enamel e.
   respiratory e.
   sulcular e.
epiturbinate
epitympanic
   recess, e. (EPR)
   space, e.
epitympanum
epoxy resin
EPR (epitympanic recess)
Epstein
   disease, E.
   pearls, E.
Epstein-Barr virus
epulides (pl. of epulis)

epulis (pl. epulides)
   congenital e.
   fibromatosa, e.
   fissurata, e.
   giant cell e.
   gigantocellularis, e.
   granulomatosa, e.
   newborn, e. of
epulofibroma
epuloid
Equen-Neuffer knife
equilibration
   ataxia, e.
equilibratory
   ataxia, e.
equilibrium
ERA (evoked response audiometry)
eraser cautery
erasion
Erczy procedure
Erhard test
Erhardt speculum
Erich
   arch bar, E.
   arch malleable bar, E.
   facial fracture appliance, E.
   facial fracture frame, E.
   forceps, E.
   laryngeal biopsy forceps, E.
   maxillary splint, E.
   nasal splint, E
   otoplasty, E.
Erich-Winter arch bar
erode
erosion
   dental e.
erosive esophagitis
errhine
eructation
erupted tooth
eruption
   active e.
   continuous e.
   delayed e.
   passive e.
   tooth e.

eruption cyst
eruptive
　gingivitis, e.
　stage, e.
erysipelas
erysipelatous
erythema
　multiforme, e.
erythematopultaceous stomatitis
erythematous
　tonsillitis, e.
erythredema polyneuropathy
erythroblastosis
　fetalis, e.
erythrodontia
erythroplakia
erythroplasia
　Queyrat, e. of
erythroprosopalgia
Escherich sign
ESD (esophagus, stomach, and duodenum)
Eska-Herrmann device
Esmarch procedure
ESI laryngoscope
esoethmoiditis
esophagalgia
esophageal
　achalasia, e.
　acid infusion test, e.
　adventitia, e.
　anastomosis, e.
　A-ring, e.
　atresia, e.
　axis, e.
　balloon, e.
　biopsy, e.
　bougie, e.
　bougienage, e.
　bougie, e.
　B-ring, e.
　bypass, e.
　cardiogram, e.
　dilatation, e.
　dilation, e.
　dilator, e.

esophageal *(continued)*
　diverticulectomy, e.
　diverticulum, e.
　duplication, e.
　dysmotility, e.
　fistula, e.
　forceps, e.
　glands, e.
　groove, e.
　hiatus, e.
　inlet, e.
　introitus, e.
　lip, e.
　lumen, e.
　lung, e.
　manometry, e.
　motility, e.
　mucosal ring, e.
　muscular ring, e.
　muscularis propria, e.
　motility, e.
　myotomy, e.
　nerves, e.
　obturator airway, e.
　obstruction, e.
　perforation, e.
　pill electrode, e.
　plexus, e.
　prosthesis, e.
　reconstruction, e.
　reflux, e.
　resection, e.
　retractor, e.
　ring, e.
　rupture, e.
　scissors, e.
　sclerosis, e.
　shears, e.
　shunt, e.
　sound, e.
　spasm, e.
　speculum, e.
　speech, e.
　sphincter, e.
　stenosis, e.
　stent, e.

esophageal *(continued)*
   stricture, e.
   tampon, e.
   tamponade, e.
   transit time, e. (ETT)
   tube, e.
   tumor, e.
   ulcer, e.
   variceal bleed, e.
   varices, e.
   vestibule, e.
   web, e.
esophagectasia
esophagectasis
esophagectomy
esophagism
esophagismus
esophagitis
   chronic peptic e.
   corrosive e.
   dissecans superficialis, e.
   erosive e.
   infectious e.
   monilial e.
   peptic e.
   reflux e.
esophagobronchial
esophagocardiomyotomy
esophagocele
esophagocologastrostomy
esophagocoloplasty
esophagoduodenostomy
esophagodynia
esophagoenterostomy
esophagoesophagostomy
esophagofundopexy
esophagogastrectomy
esophagogastric (EG)
   junction, e. (EGJ)
esophagogastroanastomosis
esophagogastroduodenoscopy (EGD)
esophagogastromyotomy
esophagogastropexy
esophagogastroplasty
esophagogastroscopy
esophagogastrostomy

esophagogram
esophagography
esophagoileostomy
esophagojejunogastrostomosis
esophagojejunogastrostomy
esophagojejunoplasty
esophagojejunostomy
esophagolaryngectomy
esophagology
esophagomalacia
esophagometer
esophagomycosis
esophagomyotomy
esophagopharynx
esophagoplasty
esophagopleural
   fistula, e.
esophagoplication
esophagoptosia
esophagoptosis
esophagorespiratory
esophagosalivary
   reflex, e.
esophagoscope
   flexible e.
   rigid e.
esophagoscopic
   cannula, e.
   catheter, e.
esophagoscopy
esophagospasm
esophagostenosis
esophagostoma
esophagostomal
   hernia, e.
esophagostomiasis
esophagostomy
esophagotome
esophagotomy
esophagotracheal
esophagram
   Besey e.
esophagraphy
esophagus
   abdominal e.
   Barrett e.

esophagus *(continued)*
   cervical e.
   corkscrew e.
   nutcracker e.
   thoracic e.
espundia
essential asthma
Esser graft
Essig
   -type splint, E.
   wiring, E.
established airway
esthesioneuroblastoma
Estlander
   cheiloplasty, E.
   flap, E.
ET (endotracheal or eustachian tube)
etching
   acid e.
ETF (eustachian tube function)
ETH (elixir terpin hydrate)
ether bronchitis
ethmocranial angle
ethmofrontal
ethmography
ethmoid
   bone, e.
   bulla, e.
   crest, e.
   fossa, e.
   plate, e.
   process, e.
ethmoidal
   air cells, e.
   angle, e.
   antrum, e.
   bone, e.
   bulla, e.
   canal, e.
   chisel, e.
   concha, e.
   crest, e.
   curette, e.
   -cutting forceps, e.
   elevator, e.
   exenteration forceps, e.

ethmoidal *(continued)*
   fissure, e.
   fossa, e.
   infundibulum, e.
   labyrinth, e.
   lamina cribrosa, e.
   nerve, e.
   notch, e.
   perpendicular plate of e.
   plate, e.
   process of Macalister, e.
   punch, e.
   sine, e.
   sinus, e.
   spine, e.
   uncinate process of e.
   vertical plate of e.
ethmoidectomy
ethmoiditis
ethmoidotomy
ethmolacrimal
ethmomaxillary
ethmonasal
ethmopalatal
ethmosphenoid
ethmoturbinal
ethmovomerine
   plate, e.
ethmyphitis
ETH/C (elixir terpin hydrate with codeine)
ETP (eustachian tube pressure)
ETT (esophageal transit time)
Etymotic ER-10A probe
eugenic acid
eugenol
eugnathia
Eulenberg disease
eunuchoid voice
eurygnathism
eustachian
   applicator, e.
   attachment, e.
   bougie, e.
   bur, e.
   canal, e.

eustachian *(continued)*
   cartilage, e.
   catheter, e.
   probe, e.
   sound, e.
   tonsil, e.
   tube, e. (ET)
   tube function, e. (ETF)
   tube pressure, e. (ETP)
   valve, e.
eustachianography
eustachitis
eustachium
euthymic
euthyroid
euthyroidism
Eves
   tonsillar knife, E.
   tonsillar snare, E.
Eves-Neivert tonsillar snare
Everclear laryngeal mirror
Eversbusch ptosis operation
evoked
   auditory response, e. (EAR)
   response audiometry, e. (ERA)
Ewald law
Ewing sign
exanthematous
excavation
excavator
   dental e.
excavator spoon
excernent
excochleation
excursion
   lateral e.
   protrusive e.
   retrusive e.
excursive
exenterate
exenteration
exfoliatio
   areata linguae, e.
Exirel
exodontia
exodontics

exodontist
exodontologist
exodontology
exognathia
exognathion
exophthalmic goiter
exophytic
exostosis
expansion
   maxillary e.
   wax e.
expansion of arch
expansion plate appliance
expectorant
   liquefying e.
   stimulant e.
   Stokes e.
expectorate
expectoration
expiratory wheezing
explorer
   dental e.
expressive aphasia
expressive-receptive aphasia
expressor
   tonsil e.
expulsion
expulsive
   coughing, e.
   gingivitis, e.
extended blepharoplasty
extension
   ridge e.
external
   auditory canal, e. (EAC)
   auditory meatus, e. (EAM)
   biphase pin fixation, e.
   ear, e.
   ear canal, e.
   ethmoidectomy, e.
   frontal sinusotomy, e.
   nasal splint, e.
   otitis media, e.
   pin fixation, e.
   sinusotomy, e.
extirpation

extra-alveolar crown
extrabronchial
extrabuccal
extraction
   dental e.
extractor
   dental e.
   esophageal e.
   tube e.
   tympanum e.
extradural
extramastoiditis
extramaxillary anchorage
extranodal
extraocular muscles (EOM)
extraocular muscles intact (EOMI)
extraoral
   anchorage, e.
   appliance, e.
extrapulmonary cough
extratracheal
extratympanic
extrinsic
   asthma, e.
   tongue muscle, e.
extrude
extrusion
exuberant
exudate
exudation
exudative
   angina, e.
   bronchitis, e.
   otitis media, e.
   tonsillitis, e.
exuviation
eye tooth
eye-ear plane

Additional entries

F

face
    adenoid f.
    bovine f.
    cleft f.
    cow f.
    dish f.
    dished f.
    frog f.
    hippocratic f.
    moon f.
    moon-shaped f.
face-lift
    procedure, f.
    scissors, f.
faceometer
face-bow
    adjustable axis f.
    kinematic f.
    transfer, f.
faceometer
faceometry
facial
    angle, f.
    appliance, f.
    asymmetry, f.
    axis, f.
    bones, f.
    branch, f.
    canal, f.
    canal hiatus, f.
    center, f.
    cleft, f.
    deformity, f.
    diplegia, f.
    droop, f.
    eminence, f.
    fracture, f.
    fracture appliance, f.
    hemihypertrophy, f.
    index, f.
    lymph nodes, f.
    nerve, f.
    nerve knife, f.

facial *(continued)*
    nerve stimulator, f.
    nevus, f.
    paralysis, f.
    plane, f.
    plethora, f.
    prosthesis, f.
    ridge, f.
    root, f.
    series, f.
    spasm, f.
    triangle, f.
facies
    adenoid f.
    Andy Gump f.
    bovine f.
    cushingoid f.
    leonine f.
    leprechaun f.
    moon f.
    moon-shaped f.
    poker f.
    Potter f.
    scaphoid f.
    steroid f.
facing
faciobrachial
faciocardiomelic dysplasia
faciocephalalgia
faciocervical
faciolingual
facioplasty
facioplegia
facioscapulohumeral
faciostenosis
Falcao suction dissector
falling palate
fallopian
    aqueduct, f.
    canal, f.
Fallopius
    aqueduct of F.
false

false *(continued)*
    anodontia, f.
    cord, f.
    croup, f.
    teeth, f.
    vocal cords, f.
fang
Farabeuf triangle
farad
faradic
Farlow
    tongue depressor, F.
    tonsil snare, F.
Farlow-Boettches tonsil snare, F.
Farnham nasal-cutting forceps
Farrell nasal applicator
Farrington
    nasal polyp forceps, F.
    septum forceps, F.
Farrior
    ear speculum, F.
    footplate pick, F.
    oval-window excavator, F.
    oval-window piston gouge
        excavator, F.
    raspatory, F.
Farrior-Dworacek canal chisel
Fasanella-Servat ptosis correction
    procedure
fascial
    plane, f.
    press, f.
fasciitis
fat
    bag, f.
    pad, f.
fatty ball of Bichet
fauces (pl. of faux)
    arches of f.
    isthmus of f.
    muscles of f.
    pillars of f.
Fauchard disease
faucial
    arch, f.
    carcinoma, f.

faucial *(continued)*
    cavity, f.
    eustachian catheter, f.
    lingual tonsillectomy, f. and
    reflex, f.
    tonsil, f.
    tonsillectomy, f.
faucitis
Faulkner
    antrum gouge, F.
    chisel, F.
    ethmoid curette, F.
    nasal curette, F.
    trocar, F.
Fauvel laryngeal forceps
faux (pl. fauces)
faveolate
feeding tube
Fein
    antrum trocar, F.
    antrum trocar needle, F.
Feldman lip retractor
feldspar
Feldstein blepharoplasty clip
fenestra (pl. fenestrae)
    cochlea, f. of
    cochleae, f. (round window)
    nov-ovalis, f.
    ovalis, f. (oval window)
    rotunda, f. (round window)
    vestibuli, f. (oval window)
fenestrae (pl. of fenestra)
fenestral
    otosclerosis, f.
fenestrated
    tracheostomy tube, f.
fenestrater
    Rosen f.
fenestration
Fergus technique
Ferguson mouth gag
Ferguson-Ackland mouth gag
Ferguson-Brophy mouth gag
Ferguson-Gwathmey mouth gag
Fergusson
    excision of maxilla, F.

Fergusson *(continued)*
  incision, F.
  operation, F.
fern leaf tongue
Ferrein
  canal, F.
  cords, F.
Ferris-Robb tonsil knife
Ferris Smith
  forceps, F.
  procedure, F.
Ferris Smith-Gruenwald sphenoid punch
Ferris Smith-Halle sinus bur
Ferris Smith-Kerrison forceps
Ferris Smith-Sewall retractor
FESS (functional endoscopic sinus surgery)
festoon
fetal alcohol syndrome
fetid
fetor
  ex ore, f.
  oris, f.
Feuerstein myringotomy tube
fever
  blister, f.
  unknown origin, f. of (FUO)
Fevre-Languepin syndrome
fiber
  alveolar f's
  alveolar crest f's
  apical f's
  cemental f's
  cementoalveolar f's
  circular f's
  dentinal f's
  dentinogenic f's
  gingival f's
  gingivodental f's
  Gottstein f's
  horizontal f's
  Korff f's
  oblique f's
  principal f's
  Prussak f's
  radiating f's of eardrum

fiber *(continued)*
  Rasmussen nerve f's
  Sappey f's
  Tomes f.
fiberoptic
  bronchoscope, f.
  bronchoscopy, f.
  esophagoscope, f.
  esophagoscopy, f.
  laryngoscope, f.
  laryngoscopy, f.
fiberscope
fiber-illuminated
Fibrel gelatin matrix implant
fibril
  dentinal f's
  Ebner f's
  Tomes f.
fibrin glue
fibrinous bronchitis
fibroadenoma
fibroamelobastic
  dentinoma, d.
  odontoma, d.
fibroangioma
fibrobronchitis
fibrocartilage
fibrocartilaginous
fibrocyst
fibroma
  ameloblastic f.
  cementifying f.
  juvenile nasopharyngeal f.
  odontogenic f.
fibromatoid
fibromatosis
  colli, f.
  gingivae, f.
  gingival f.
fibromatous
fibromectomy
fibromembranous
fibromyalgia
fibro-osseous
  otitis media, f.
fibro-osteoma

fibroplasia
fibroplastic
fibropurulent
fibrosarcoma
fibrosclerosis
fibrosis
fibrositis
fibrous union
Fick perforation of footplate
fifth cranial nerve
fila (pl. of filum)
file
filiform
    papillae of tongue, f.
filled tooth
filling
    complex f.
    composite f.
    compound f.
    direct f.
    direct resin f.
    ditched f.
    gold f.
    indirect f.
    permanent f.
    porcelain f.
    retrograde f.
    reverse f.
    root canal f.
    root-end f.
    silver f.
    temporary f.
    treatment f.
film
    bite-wing f.
    lateral jaw f.
    occlusal f.
    periapical f.
    plain f.
    spot f.
    x-ray f.
filmy tongue
filtrum ventriculi
filum (pl. fila)
fimbriae of tongue
fine-needle

fine-needle *(continued)*
    aspiration, f. (FNA)
    aspiration biopsy (FNAB)
    aspiration cytology (FNAC)
finger
    cot, f.
    dissection, f.
    spelling, f.
    spring, f.
Fink laryngoscope
Finnoff laryngoscope
firing
    needle, f.
    turbinates, f. of
first
    arch syndrome, f.
    cranial nerve, f.
    pharyngeal pouch, f.
Fish
    nasal forceps, F.
    sinus probe, F.
Fisher
    dissector, F.
    tonsil dissector, F.
    tonsil knife, F.
Fischgold bimastoid line
fissura (pl. fissurae)
    antitragohelicina, f.
fissurae (pl. of fissura)
fissural cyst
fissure
    auricular f.
    branchial f's
    craniofacial f.
    enamel f.
    entorbital f.
    ethmoid f.
    glaserian f.
    glottis, f. of
    inferior orbital f.
    intratonsillar f.
    lacrimal f.
    mandibular f's
    maxillary f.
    occipitosphenoidal f.
    oral f.

fissure *(continued)*
   orbital f.
   palpebral f.
   parietosphenoid f.
   petromastoid f.
   petrosphenoidal f.
   petrosquamosal f.
   petrotympanic f.
   pterygomaxillary f.
   pterygopalatine f.
   pterygotympanic f.
   Santorini f's
   sphenoidal f.
   sphenomaxillary f.
   sphenooccipital f.
   sphenopetrosal f.
   squamotympanic f.
   tonsillar f.
   tympanic f.
   tympanomastoid f.
   tympanosquamous f.
   zygomaticosphenoid f.
fissure bur
fissure cavity
fissured
   fracture, f.
   tongue, f.
fistula test
fistula (pl. fistulae)
   auris congenita, f.
   branchial f.
   cibalis, f.
   colli congenita, f.
   craniosinus f.
   esophagopleural f.
   Gross tracheoesophageal f.
   lacrimal f.
   oroantral f.
   parotid f.
   perilymph f.
   pharyngeal f.
   preauricular f.
   salivary f.
   submental f.
   thyroglossal f.
   tracheal f.

fistula (pl. fistulae) *(continued)*
   tracheoesophageal f.
   tracheoinnominate f.
fistulae (pl. of fistula)
fistula hook
fistulatome
fistulectomy
fistulization
fistulotomy
fistulous
   tract, f.
fixation nystagmus
fixed
   appliance, f.
   partial denture, f.
Flagg laryngoscope
flange
Flannery ear speculum
flap
   skin f.
   tympanomeatal f.
flap harvest
flap operation
flap was swung
flaring
   alar f.
   nostrils, f. of
flask
   casting f.
   crown f.
   denture f.
   refractory f.
flasking
flat
   affect, f.
   face, f.
   lip, f.
   nose, f.
   tongue, f.
flattening
   nasolabial fold, f. of
Fleischmann
   bursa, F.
   follicle, F.
Fletcher tonsil knife
fletcherism

fleur-de-lis forehead flap
flexible fiberoptic bronchoscopy
floating tooth
floor
   mouth, f. of
   nose, f. of
flora
   mixed common f.
   normal f.
   oral f.
florid
floss
flossing
Flouren law
Flower index
fluent aphasia
fluffy-cuffed tube
flunisolide
fluoridation
fluoride
   stannous f.
fluoridize
fluorination
fluorine
fluoroscopy
fluorosis
fluroapatite
flush
   malar f.
flux
fluxion
flying
   baby bird incision, f.
   -bird incision, f.
   wing incision, f.
FNA (fine-needle aspiration)
FNAB (fine-needle aspiration biopsy)
FNAC (fine-needle aspiration cytology)
foam embolus
Foerster system
foil
   cohesive gold f.
   gold f.
   mat f.
   platinum f.
   tin f.

foil passer
foil pellet
fold
   alar f's
   aryepiglottic f.
   aryepiglottic f. of Collier
   epicanthal f.
   glossoepiglottic f.
   Hasner f.
   incudal f.
   lacrimal f.
   mallear f.
   mucobuccal f.
   mucolabial f.
   mucosal f.
   mucosobuccal f.
   nasolabial f.
   nasopharyngeal f.
   palatine f's
   palpebral f.
   palpebronasal f.
   pharyngoepiglottic f.
   salpingopalatine f.
   salpingopharyngeal f.
   stapedial f.
   sublingual f.
   ventricular f. of larynx
   vestibular f.
   vocal f.
folding laryngoscope
folia (pl. of folium)
folian process
folium (pl. folia)
   lingual f.
Follius
   muscle, F.
   process, F.
follicle
   dental f.
   Fleischmann f.
   laryngeal lymphatic f's
   lingual f's
   lymphatic f's of tongue
   nasal mucous f's
   thyroid f's
   tooth f.

follicular
    bronchiectasis, f.
    pharyngitis, f.
    stomatitis, f.
    tonsillitis, f.
folliculi (pl. of folliculus)
folliculitis
folliculus (pl. folliculi)
Fomon
    chisel, F.
    knife, F.
    nasal rasp, F.
    nostril elevator, F.
    otoplasty, F.
    periosteotome, F.
    raspatory, F.
    retractor, F.
    scissors, F.
fontanelle
fonticuli (pl. of fonticulus)
fonticulus (pl. fonticuli)
food
    asthma, f.
    bolus, f.
foot-and-mouth disease
footplate
    stapes, f. of
foramen (pl. foramina)
    accessory f.
    alveolar f. of maxilla
    apical f.
    auditory f.
    caecum linguae, f.
    caroticotympanic f.
    condyloid f.
    cribroethmoid f.
    dental f.
    esophageal f.
    ethmoidal f.
    external auditory f.
    frontoethmoid f.
    glandular f. of Morgagni
    glandular f. of tongue
    Huschke f.
    hypoglossal f.
    incisive f.

foramen (pl. foramina) *(continued)*
    incisivum, f.
    infraorbital f.
    internal auditory f.
    jugular f.
    malar f.
    mandibular f.
    mastoid f.
    mastoideum, f.
    maxillary f.
    mental f.
    nasal f.
    olfactory f.
    orbitomalar f.
    ovale, f.
    palatine f.
    pterygopalatine f.
    radicis dentis, f.
    rivinian, f.
    Rivinus f.
    root f.
    rotundum ossis sphenoidalis, f.
    Scarpa, f. of
    Scarpa f.
    singulare, f.
    sphenopalatine f.
    sphenopalatinum, f.
    Spondel f.
    Stensen, f. of
    Stensen f.
    stylomastoid f.
    stylomastoideum, f.
    supraorbital f.
    temporomalar f.
    thyroid f.
    tonsillar f.
    zygomatic f.
    zygomaticofacial f.
    zygomatic-orbital f.
    zygomaticotemporal f.
foramina (pl. of foramen)
foraminal
    node, f.
    stenosis, f.
foraminotomy
force

force *(continued)*
    chewing f.
    extraoral f.
    masticatory f.
    occlusal f.
    reciprocal f.
Fordyce granules
Foregger
    bronchoscope, F.
    laryngoscope, F.
    rigid esophagoscope, F.
forehead
foreign body
    aspirated f.
    metallic f.
    swallowed f.
foreign body aspiration
foreign body impaction
foreign body sensation
forensic dentistry
forked tongue
form
    arch f.
    retention f.
    spherical f. of occlusion
    tooth f.
fornices (pl. of fornix)
fornix (pl. fornices)
    pharyngis, f.
    pharynx, f. of
formula
    Seiler f.
Foroblique esophagoscope
Forrester cervical collar brace
Forschheimer spots
fossa (pl. fossae)
    amygdaloid f.
    articular f.
    canine f.
    cochleariform f.
    condylar f.
    condyloid f.
    digastric f.
    ethmoid f.
    incisive f.
    incudis, f.

fossa (pl. fossae) *(continued)*
    infratemporal f.
    lacrimal f.
    Malgaigne f.
    mandibular f.
    mastoid f.
    maxillary f.
    mylohyoid f.
    myrtiform f.
    nasal f.
    navicular f. of Cruveilhier
    olfactory f.
    oral f.
    pharyngeal f.
    pharyngomaxillary f.
    piriform f.
    prenasal f.
    pterygoid f.
    pterygomaxillary f.
    pterygopalatine f.
    retromandibular f.
    Rosenmuller, f. of
    scaphoid f.
    sphenomaxillary f.
    sublingual f.
    submandibular f.
    submaxillary f.
    subnasal f.
    subpyramidal f.
    supratonsillar f.
    tonsillar f.
    triangular f. of auricle
    triangularis, f.
    trochlear f.
    vestibular f.
    zygomatic f.
fossae (pl. of fossa)
fossula (pl. fossulae)
fossulae (pl. of fossula)
fossulate
Foster-Ballenger
    forceps, F.
    nasal speculum, F.
Fothergill
    disease, F.
    neuralgia, F.

Fothergill *(continued)*
   sore throat, F.
foundation
   denture f.
four
   -day syndrome, f.
   -flap cleft palate repair, f.
   -flap palatoplasty, f.
   -handed dentistry, f.
   -tailed bandage, f.
Fournier teeth
fourth
   cranial nerve, f.
   pharyngeal pouch, f.
fovea (pl. foveae)
foveae (pl. of fovea)
foveate
foveation
Fowler test
Fox
   scissors, F.
   splint, F.
fracture
   appliance, f.
   fragment, f.
fractured
   tooth, f.
   windpipe, f.
Fraenkel
   appliance, F.
   forceps, F.
   glands, F.
   sinus probe, F.
   speculum, F.
   test, F.
Fragen anterior commissure microlaryngoscope
fragile X syndrome
Franceschetti syndrome
Franceschetti-Jadassohn syndrome
Francois syndrome
Frankel appliance
Frankfort Horizontal plane
franklinic taste
Frazier
   nasal suction tip, F.

Frazier *(continued)*
   tube, F.
Frazier-Paparella mastoid tube
Frazier-Spiller operation
free
   gingiva, f.
   graft, f.
   gum, f.
   thyroxine index, f. (FTI)
Freeman modification of Bernard-Burrows procedure
Freeman-Sheldon syndrome
Freer
   chisel, F.
   elevator, F.
   hook, F.
   knife, F.
   nasal gouge, F.
   nasoseptal elevator, F.
   submucous retractor, F.
Freer-Ingal
   septal knife, S.
   submucous knife, S.
freeway space
freeze
   -dried, f.
   -drying, f.
Freimuth ear curette
fremitus
   bronchial f.
   tussive f.
   vocal f.
frena (pl. of frenum)
frenal
French flap
French-pattern lacrimal probe
Frenckner intrapetrosal drainage procedure
frenectomy
frenoplasty
frenotomy
   lingual f.
frenula (pl. of frenulum)
frenulectomy
frenuloplasty
frenulum (pl. frenula)

frenulum (pl. frenula) *(continued)*
    labii inferioris, f.
    labii superioris, f.
    linguae, f.
    lip, f. of
    tongue, f. of
frenum (pl. frena)
    labiorum, f.
    lingual, f.
Frenzel ear operating head
Fresgen frontal sinus probe
fressreflex
Frey syndrome
fricative
frictional clip
Friedenwald ptosis operation
Friedenwald-Guyton technique
Friedmann vasomotor syndrome
Friedreich
    ataxia, F.
    tabes, F.
Friesner
    ear knife, F.
    ear perforator, F.
Frigitronics cryoprobe
frit
frog
    breathing, f.
    face, f.
Frohm mouth gag
frontad
frontal
    air sinuses, f.
    axis, f.
    bone, f.
    lobe, f.
    process of maxilla, f.
    recess, f.
    sinus, f.
    sinusotomy, f.
frontalis
frontipetal
frontocortical aphasia
frontoethmoidal
frontolacrimal
frontolenticular aphasia

frontomalar
frontomaxillary
frontomental diameter
frontonasal
    duct, f.
    dysplasia, f.
    process, f.
fronto-occipital
frontoparietal
frontosphenoidal
frontotemporal
frontozygomatic
Froschel symptom
frostbite
frostbitten
frothy sputum
Fry nasal forceps
FSR (fusiform skin revision)
FTI (free thyroxine index)
Fuchs position
Fujinon flexible bronchoscope
fulcrum line
fulguration
full
    denture, f.
    -lumen esophagoscope, f.
    -veneer crown, f.
Fulton mouth gag
functional
    aphasia, f.
    chew-in record, f.
    deafness, f.
    endoscopic sinus surgery, f. (FESS)
fundi (pl. of fundus)
fundoplication
fundus (pl. fundi)
fungal
fungate
fungating
fungi (pl. of fungus)
fungiform
    papillae, f.
fungoid
fungous
fungus (pl. fungi)
FUO (fever of unknown origin)

furca
furcal
furcation
furcula
furious rabies
Furniss otoplasty
furred tongue
furrow
furrowed
   brow, f.
   tongue, f.
furry teeth
furuncle
furuncular
   otitis, f.
furunculosis
fused teeth
fusiform
   fossa, f.
fusion
fusospirillary
fusospirillosis
fusospirochetal
   gingivitis, f.
   stomatitis, f.

Additional entries

G

G (gingival)
Gabarro graft
gadolinium
gag
    mouth g.
gag reflex
gagging
galeal-pericranial flap
Galen anastomosis
Galezowski lacrimal dilator
Gallagher antral frontal raspatory
galoche chin
GALT (gut-associated lymphoid tissue)
galvanic
    nystagmus, g.
    vertigo, g.
galvanism
galvanization
galvanocautery
galvanochemical
galvanogustometer
Gandhi knife
ganglia (pl. of ganglion)
ganglial
ganglioglioma
ganglion (pl. ganglia)
    acousticofacial g.
    Andersch g.
    Arnold auricular g.
    auricular g.
    Blandin g.
    Bochdalek g.
    carotid g.
    Cloquet g.
    cochlear g.
    Corti g.
    Ehrenritter g.
    geniculate g.
    geniculi nervi facialis, g.
    glossopharyngeal, g. of
    jugular g. of glossopharyngeal nerve
    Kuttner g.
    lesser g. of Meckel

ganglion (pl. ganglia) *(continued)*
    lower g. of glossopharyngeal nerve
    Meckel g.
    Muller, g. of
    nodose g.
    olfactory g.
    otic g.
    petrosal g.
    petrous g.
    pharyngeal g.
    pterygopalatine g.
    Scarpa g.
    Schmiedel g.
    sphenomaxillary g.
    sphenopalatine g.
    spiral g.
    spiral g. of cochlea
    sublingual g.
    submandibular g.
    submaxillary g.
    trigeminal g.
    tympanic g.
    tympanic g. of Valentin
    Valentin g.
    vestibular g.
ganglionectomy
ganglionic saliva
ganglionitis
gangosa
gangrene
gangrenous
    pharyngitis, g.
    stomatitis, g.
gap
    air-bone g.
    interocclusal g.
gap arthroplasty
Gardiner-Brown tuning fork
Gardner syndrome
Garel sign
Garfield-Holinger laryngoscope
gargarism
gargle

gargling
garnet
gasp
Gasser ganglion
gasserian ganglion
gastroesophageal (GE)
    reflux, g. (GER)
    reflux disease, g. (GERD)
    regurgitation, g.
gastroesophagitis
gastroesophagostomy
Gault
    cochleopalpebral reflex, G.
    test, G.
gauze
    pack, g.
    wick, g.
Gavallo earlobe procedure
Gayet technique
gaze nystagmus
GBA (gingivobuccoaxial)
GCA (giant cell arteritis)
GCS (Glasgow Coma Scale)
GE (gastroesophageal)
    reflux, G.
gear
    cervical g.
    head g.
Gegenbaur's sulcus
Gelfilm
    myringoplasty, G.
    stent, G.
Gelfoam
    pledget, G.
    sponge, G.
Gell and Coombs classification
Gelle test
geminate tooth
gemination
gena
genal
    gland, g.
    line, g.
Gendelach sphenoid punch
genetic deafness
genial apophysis

geniocheiloplasty
genioglossal
genioglossus
geniohyoglossus
geniohyoid
geniohyoideus
genion
geniomandibular
    groove, g.
genioplasty
genu (pl. genua)
genua (pl. of genu)
genyantralgia
genyantritis
genyantrum
genycheiloplasty
genyplasty
Georgiade
    halo apparatus, G.
    intraoral traction, G.
geographic tongue
Gerber stud
GER (gastroesophageal reflux)
GERD (gastroesophageal reflux disease)
Gerdy
    hyoid fossa, G.
    interauricular loop, G.
Gerhardt syndrome
Gerhardt-Semon law
Gerlach tonsil
Gerlier disease
germ
    dental g.
    enamel g.
    tooth g.
German measles
germinal
    center, g.
gerodontia
gerodontics
gerodontist
gerodontology
Gersuny otoplasty
Gerzog
    ear knife, G.
    hammer, G.

Gerzog *(continued)*
    mastoid mallet, G.
    speculum, G.
Gerzog-Ralks ear knife
gesticulatory tic
geumaphobia
Gey solution
GG or S (glands, goiter, or stiffness)
Gherini-Kauffman endo-otoprobe
giant cell
    arteritis, g. (GCA)
    reparative granuloma, g.
gibberish aphasia
giddiness
giddy
Gifford mastoid retractor
Gifford-Jansen mastoid retractor
Gigli wire saw
Gill cleft palate elevator
Gilles de la Tourette syndrome
Gillies
    approach, G.
    graft, G.
    hook, G.
    operation, G.
    suture, G.
    zygomatic arch fracture procedure, G.
    zygomatic hook, G.
Gillies-Dingman hook
Gilmer
    intermaxillary fixation, G.
    tooth splint, g.
    wiring, G.
gingiva (pl. gingivae)
    alveolar g.
    areolar g.
    attached g.
    buccal g.
    cemental g.
    free g.
    interdental g.
    interproximal g.
    labial g.
    lingual g.
    marginal g.
    papillary g.

gingiva (pl. gingivae) *(continued)*
    septal g.
    unattached g.
gingivae (pl. of gingiva)
gingival (G)
    abscess, g.
    cartilage, g.
    clamp, g.
    cleft, g.
    contour, g.
    crest, g.
    crevice, g.
    cuff, g.
    denture contour, g.
    epithelium, g.
    festoon, g.
    glands, g.
    incision, g.
    lamina propria, g.
    lancet, g.
    line, g.
    margin, g.
    recession, g.
    stippling, g.
    sulcus, g.
    trough, g.
gingivalgia
gingivally
gingivectomy
gingivitis
    acute necrotizing ulcerative g.
        (ANUG)
    acute ulceromembranous g.
    atrophic senile g.
    bismuth g.
    catarrhal g.
    cotton-roll g.
    desquamative g.
    Dilantin g.
    diphenylhydantoin g.
    eruptive g.
    expulsive g.
    fusospirochetal g.
    gravidum, g.
    hemorrhagic g.
    herpetic g.

gingivitis *(continued)*
   hormonal g.
   hyperplastic g.
   interstitial g.
   marginal g.
   necrotizing ulcerative g.
   papillary g.
   phagedenic g.
   pregnancy g.
   scorbutic g.
   senile atrophic g.
   suppurative marginal g.
   tuberculous g.
   ulceromembranous g.
   Vincent g.
gingivoaxial
gingivobuccal
gingivobuccoaxial (GBA)
gingivoglossitis
gingivolabial (GLA)
gingivolinguoaxial (GLA)
gingivoperiodontitis
   necrotizing ulcerative g.
gingivoplasty
gingivosis
gingivostomatitis
   acute necrotizing ulcerative g. (ANUG)
   herpetic g.
Giralde procedure
GLA (gingivolabial or gingivolinguoaxial)
glabella
glabellad
glabellar
glabelloalveolar
glabellomeatal line
glabellum
gland
   admaxillary g.
   arytenoid g's
   auricular g.
   Bauhin g.'s
   Blandin g's
   Blandin and Nuhn g's
   Bowman g's

gland *(continued)*
   bronchial g's
   buccal g's
   carotid g.
   ceruminous g's
   cheek g's
   Ciaccio g's
   Cobelli g's
   Ebner g's
   esophageal g's
   follicular g's of tongue
   Fraenkel g's
   genal g.
   gingival g's
   Gley g's
   glossopalatine g's
   gustatory g's
   Harder g's
   harderian g's
   Henle g's
   jugular g's
   Krause g's
   labial g's
   lacrimal g.
   lingual g's
   malar g's
   molar g's
   muciparous g's
   mucous g's
   Nuhn g's
   olfactory g's
   palatine g's
   palpebral g's
   parathyroid g's
   parotid g.
   pharyngeal g's
   Poirier g's
   prehyoid g's
   retrolingual g.
   retromolar g.
   Rivinus g.
   Rosenmuller g.
   salivary g.
   Sandstrom g's
   seromucous g.
   Serres g's

gland *(continued)*
    Stahr g.
    staphyline g's
    subauricular g's
    sublingual g.
    submandibular g.
    submaxillary g.
    Suzanne g.
    thyroid g.
    tongue, g's of
    tracheal g.
    tympanic g's
    Waldeyer g's
    Weber g's
    Wolfring, g's of
    Zeis, g's of
    Zuckerkandl g.
Glandosane
glandula (pl. glandulae)
glandulae (pl. of glandula)
glandular
glandule
glaserian
    artery, g.
    fissure, g.
Glasgow Coma Scale (GCS)
glass
    -blowers' mouth, g.
    ionomer cement, g.
    jaw, g.
Glasscock ear dressing
Glatzel mirror
glaze
Gleason raspatory
glenoid fossa
Gley glands
glide
    mandibular g.
    occlusal g.
gliding movement
glioma
Glisson capsule
global aphasia
globoid
globose
globular

globule
globulomaxillary
globus
    hystericus, g.
glomangioma
glomeruli (pl. of glomerulus)
glomerulus (pl. glomeruli)
glomus
    jugulare, g.
    tympanicum, g.
Glori post-keloid surgery pressure earrings
glossa
glossagra
glossal
glossalgia
glossanthrax
glossectomy
glossitis
    areata exfoliativa, g.
    atrophic g.
    benign migratory g.
    desiccans, g.
    Hunter g.
    idiopathic g.
    median rhomboid g.
    migrans, g.
    Moeller g.
    parasitica, g.
    psychogenic g.
    rhomboid g.
    rhomboidea mediana, g.
glossocele
glossocoma
glossodynamometer
glossodynia
    exfoliativa, g.
glossoepiglottic
glossoepiglottidean
    folds, g.
    ligament, g.
glossograph
glossohyal
glossokinesthetic
glossolabial
glossolalia

glossology
glossolysis
glossolytic
glossomantia
glossoncus
glossopalatine
   arch, g.
   glands, g.
   muscle, g.
   sulcus, g.
glossopalatinus
glossopathy
glossopexy
glossopharyngeal
   breathing, g.
   nerve, g.
   neuralgia, g.
   neurotomy, g.
   sympathetic afferent fibers, g.
glossopharyngeum
glossopharyngeus
glossophobia
glossophytia
glossoplasty
glossoplegia
glossoptosis
glossopyrosis
glossorrhaphy
glossoscopy
glossospasm
glossosteresis
glossotilt
glossotomy
glossotrichia
glottal
glottic
   atresia, g.
   chink, g.
   extension, g.
   spasm, g.
   stop, g.
glottides (pl. of glottis)
glottis (pl. glottides)
   false g.
   intercartilaginous g.
   respiratoria, g.

glottis (pl. glottides) *(continued)*
   respiratory g.
   true g.
   vocalis, g.
glottology
glucagonoma syndrome
glue
   -ear, g.
   sniffing, g.
gluey
glyceryl guaiacolate syrup
glycogeusia
glycosialia
glycosialorrhea
gnarled enamel
gnashing
gnathalgia
gnathic
   index, g.
gnathion
gnathitis
gnathocephalus
gnathodynamics
gnathodynamometer
gnathodynia
gnathography
gnathologic
gnathological
   occlusion procedure, g.
   splint, g.
gnathology
gnathoplasty
gnathoschisis
gnathostat
gnathostatic
   cast, g.
gnathostomiasis
goblet cells
goiter
   aberrant g.
   adenomatous g.
   Basedow g.
   colloid g.
   congenital g.
   cystic g.
   diffuse g.

goiter *(continued)*
   diving g.
   endemic g.
   exophthalmic g.
   fibrous g.
   follicular g.
   hyperplastic g.
   intrathoracic g.
   iodide g.
   lingual g.
   lymphadenoid g.
   mediastinal g.
   multinodular g.
   nodular g.
   nontoxic g.
   parenchymatous g.
   perivascular g.
   plunging g.
   retrovascular g.
   simple g.
   substernal g.
   suffocative g.
   toxic g.
   toxic multinodular g.
   vascular g.
   wandering g.
   x-ray g.
goitrogenous
goitrous
   autoimmune thyroiditis, g.
gold
   cohesive g.
   mat g.
gold alloy
gold condenser
gold crown
gold dental casting
gold ear marker
gold filling
gold foil
gold post
gold solder
gold tooth
Goldenhar syndrome
Goldman-Fox knife
Goldman-Fristoe Test of Articulation
Goldman-Kazanjian forceps
Goldman-McNeill blepharostat
Goldnamer ear basin
Goldstein
   lacrimal sac retractor, g.
   hemoptysis, G.
Goltz theory
gonial
   angle, g.
   notch, g.
gonion
gonoblast
gonococcal stomatitis
gonorrheal stomatitis
Good
   raspatory, G.
   tonsillar scissors, G.
Good-Reiner tonsil scissors
Goode
   myringotomy tube, G.
   nasal splint, G.
   T-tube, G.
   ventilation tube, G.
Goode-Magne nasal airway splint
Goodfellow frontal sinus cannula
Goodhill tonsillar forceps
Goodman syndrome
Goodyear
   tonsillar knife, G.
   uvular retractor, G.
Gorlin syndrome
Gorlin-Psaume syndrome
Gorney
   face-lift scissors, G.
   rhytidectomy scissors, G.
   septal scissors, G.
   turbinate scissors, G.
gorondou
Goslee tooth
gothic
   arch tracing, g.
   palate, g.
Gottinger line
Gottlieb epithelial attachment
Gottschalk
   middle ear aspirator, G.

Gottschalk *(continued)*
  saw, G.
Gottstein
  fibers, G.
  process, G.
gouge
gouging
goundou
gouty pearl
Gradenigo syndrome
gradient recalled acquisition in the steady state (GRASS)
Graether
  buttonhook, G.
  collar button, G.
graft
  flap g.
  free g.
  full-thickness g.
  pedicle g.
  split-thickness g.
  tube g.
graft tooth
grafting
Grancher triad
Granger line
granulation tissue
granuloma
  pyogenicum, g.
granulomatosis
  Wegener g.
granulomatous
granulosis
  rubra nasi, g.
graphomotor aphasia
Grashey aphasia
grasping forceps
GRASS (gradient recalled acquisition in the steady state)
  scan, G.
gravedo
Graves disease
Great Ormand Street
  tracheostomy, G.
  tube, G.
greater alar cartilage

green
  rhinorrhea, g.
  sputum, g.
Green mouth gag
Green-Sewall mouth gag
Greene-Vardiman-Black classification
greenstick fracture
Greisinger sign
Grimsdale technique
grinder
grinders' asthma
grinding
  -in, g.
  selective g.
  wheel, g.
grippal
grippe
Grob dysplasia linguofacialis
Groenholm lid retractor
grommet
  drain tube, g.
  tube, g.
Grondahl-Finney esophagogastroplasty
Groningen button
groove
  alveolingual g.
  branchial g.
  buccal developmental g.
  carotid g.
  dental g.
  developmental g's
  distobuccal developmental g's
  distolingual developmental g's
  enamel g's
  ethmoidal g.
  eustachian tube, g. for
  gingival g.
  infraorbital g.
  interdental g.
  labial g.
  lacrimal g.
  laryngotracheal g.
  mesiobuccal developmental g.
  mesiolingual developmental g.
  mylohyoid g.
  nasal g.

groove *(continued)*
   nasolacrimal g.
   nasomaxillary
   nasopalatine g.
   nasopharyngeal g.
   occlusal g.
   olfactory g.
   palatine g.
   palatomaxillary g.
   pharyngeal g.
   pterygopalatine g.
   sigmoid g.
   trigeminal g.
   tympanic g.
   Verga lacrimal g.
   visceral g.
   vomeral g.
grooved tongue
Gross
   curette, G.
   ear hook, G.
   ear spoon, G.
   ear spud, G.
ground glass discoloration
growth axis
Gruber
   bougies, G.
   ear speculum, G.
Gruenwald
   ear forceps, G.
   nasal-cutting forceps, G.
   nasal punch, G.
Gruenwald-Bryant forceps
grumous debris
grunting
   breath sounds, g.
   respirations, g.
Gruntzig dilating catheter
guaiacol
guaifenesin
guaithylline
guarded osteotome
gubernaculum
   dentis, g.
Gubler paralysis
Gudden atrophy

Guedel
   airway, G.
   blade, G.
   laryngoscope, G.
   laryngoscope blade, G.
   rubber airway, g.
Guerin fracture
Guggenheim adenoid forceps
Guibor canaliculus intubation set
Guidi canal
Guilford stapedectomy
guillotine
   adenotome, g.
Guinon disease
gullet
Gull-Toynbee law
gum
   blue g.
   karaya g.
   red g.
   spongy g's
   sterculia g.
gum abscess
gum bleeding
gum pads
gum polyp
gum rash
gum scissors
gum tissue
gumboil
gumline
gumma
Gundelach punch
Gunning splint
gurgling
   breath sounds, g.
   respirations, g.
gurgulio
gustation
gustatism
gustatory
   audition, g.
   bud, g.
   bulb, g.
   cell, g.
   hyperhidrosis, g.

gustatory *(continued)*
    organ, g.
    pore, g.
    receptor, g.
    sweating, g.
gustin
gustolacrimal
gustometer
gustometry
gut-associated lymphoid tissue (GALT)
Gutgeman auricular appendage clamp
Guttaform dental impression material
gutta-percha
    baseplate, g.
    cone, g.
    point, g.

gutter
    fracture, g.
gutteral
    cartilage, g.
gutterophony
gutterotetany
guttur
guttural
    voice, g.
gutturotetany
Guy model nasal gouge
Guyton technique
Guzman-Blanco epiglottis retractor
gypsum
gyrus

Additional entries

H

H-1 blocker
habenula (pl. habenulae)
habenulae (pl. of habenula)
habenular
habit
    clamping h.
    clenching h.
    masticatory h.
    oral h.
habit-breaking appliance
habit spasm
habit tic
habitus
hacking cough
Haemophilus influenzae (H-flu)
hag teeth
Hagedorn cheiloplasty
Hagedorn-LeMesurier procedure
Hagerty procedure
hair teeth
hair-bearing graft
hairline
hairy
    ears, h.
    nevus, h.
    tongue, h.
Haitz canaliculus punch
Hajek
    antral punch
    retractor H.
    septal chisel, H.
    sphenoid punch forceps, H.
Hajek-Ballenger septal elevator
Hajek-Koffler
    punch forceps, H.
    sphenoid punch, H.
Hajek-Skillern punch
Hajek-Tieck nasal speculum
half-cap crown
half-Z technique
halitosis
halitus
Hall

Hall *(continued)*
    dermatome, H.
    mastoid bur, H.
    ototome, H.
Halle
    ethmoid curette, H.
    nasal elevator, H.
    septal needle, H.
    sinus curette, H.
    speculum, H.
Halle-Tieck nasal speculum
Hallerman-Streif-Francois syndrome
Hallpike caloric stimulation test
halo traction
Haloscale respirometer
halzoun
Hamilton tongue depressor
hammer
    dental h.
hammer nose
Hammerschlag phenomenon
hammock bandage
Hamrick elevator
hamular
    process, h.
hamuli (pl. of hamulus)
hamulus (pl. hamuli)
    cochleae, h.
    lacrimalis, h.
    pterygoideus, h.
Hand-E-Vent
hand-held nebulizer
Hand-Schuller-Christian disease
H angle
handpiece
    air-bearing turbine h.
    contra-angle h.
    high-speed h.
Handtrol electrosurgical pencil
hangman's fracture
Hanhart syndrome
Hannover intermediate membrane
haplodont

Hapsburg
  jaw, H.
  lip, H.
hard palate
Harder glands
harderian glands
Hardy-Sella punch
harelip
  suture, h.
Harmon technique
harmony
  functional occlusal h.
  occlusal h.
Harold Hayes eustachian bougie
Harrington esophageal diverticulectomy
Harris migrainous neuralgia
Harrison tonsillar knife
harsh
  cough, h.
  respirations, h.
Hartel treatment
Hartley-Krause operation
Hartmann
  adenoidal curette, H.
  ear-dressing forceps, H.
  ear forceps, H.
  eustachian catheter, H.
  mastoid rongeur, H.
  nasal speculum, H.
  nasal-dressing forceps, H.
  punch, H.
  rongeur, H.
  solution, H.
  speculum, H.
  tonsillar dissector, H.
  tuning fork, H.
Hartman-Citelli ear forceps
Hartmann-Dewaxer speculum
Hartmann-Gruenwald nasal-cutting
  forceps
Hartmann-Herzfeld ear rongeur
Hartmann-Noyes nasal-dressing forceps
Hartman-Proctor ear forceps
harvest
Hasegawa-Naito procedure
Hashimoto

Hashimoto *(continued)*
  struma, H.
  thyroiditis, H.
Haslinger
  bronchoscope, H.
  esophagoscope, H.
  headrest, H.
  laryngoscope, H.
  retractor, H.
  tonsil hemostat, H.
  tracheobroncho-esophagoscope, H.
  tracheoscope, H.
  uvula retractor, H.
Hasner
  fold, H.
  valve, H.
hat-band headache
Hatchcock sign
hatchet
  enamel h.
Hauenstein right-angle screwdriver
hauptganglion of Kuttner
Haverhill
  fever, H.
  procedure, H.
haversian canal
hawk-bill incisors
Hawley
  appliance, H.
  retainer, H.
hay fever
Hayden curette
Hayton-Williams mouth gag
HD (hearing distance)
head of malleus
headache
headcap
headgear
headlight
headrest
heaped-up debris
hearing
  color h.
  double disharmonic h.
  impaired h.
  monaural h.

hearing *(continued)*
    visual h.
hearing aid
hearing deficit
hearing distance (HD)
hearing hallucinations
hearing level
hearing loss
    Alexander h.
    conductive h.
    pagetoid h.
    paradoxic h.
    sensorineural h.
    transmission h.
hearing prosthesis
hearing test
hearing threshold
hearing whistle
heat-curing resin
Heath procedure
heaves
Heberden asthma
Heerfordt syndrome
Heerman
    alligator ear forceps, H.
    chisel, H.
    gouge, H.
    incision, H.
Heffernan speculum
Heidenhaim syndrome
height
    contour, h. of
    cusp h.
    facial h.
height vertigo
Heimlich
    maneuver, H.
    sign, H.
Heiss mastoid retractor
Heister mouth gag
helical
helicoid
helicotrema
heliotrope infraorbital discoloration
Helistat
helix

Hellat sign
Heller esophagomyotomy
Heller-Belsey procedure
Heller-Nissen procedure
Helsper
    laryngectomy button, H.
    tracheostoma vent, H.
Helvetius ligament
hemangioma
Hemholtz ligament
hemiageusia
hemianacusia
hemianosmia
hemiatrophy
hemifacial
    spasm, h. (HFS)
hemigeusia
hemiglossal
hemiglossectomy
hemiglossitis
hemignathia
hemilaryngectomy
hemilingual
hemimacroglossia
hemimandibulectomy
hemimaxillectomy
hemiopalgia
hemiplegia
hemisectomy
hemitransfixion incision
hemorrhage
hemorrhagic
    bronchitis, h.
    diathesis, h.
    gingivitis, h.
hemostasis
hemostat
hemostatic
    eraser, h.
    tonsil guillotine, h.
    tonsillectome, h.
hemistrumectomy
hemotympanum
hen-cluck stertor
Henke
    space, H.

Henke *(continued)*
    tonsillar dissector, H.
Henle
    glands, H.
    spine, H.
Hennebert sign
Henner
    endaural retractor, H.
    T-model endaural retractor, H.
henpuye
Henry cilia forceps
Hensen cells
Henton
    tonsillar suture hook, H.
    tonsillar suture needle, H.
herald patch
Herbst appliance
hereditary
    brown enamel, h.
    cutaneomandibular polyoncosis, h.
    goiter and deafness, h.
    hematuria-nephropathy-deafness, h.
    opalescent dentin, h.
    thymic dysplasia, h.
Hering nerves
Hermansky-Pudlak syndrome
hernia
    esophagostomal h.
    hiatal h. (HH)
    paraesophageal h.
    sliding esophageal hiatal h.
herniated
herniation
herpangina
herpes
    catarrhalis, h.
    febrilis, h.
    labialis, h.
    oticus, h.
    simplex, h.
    zoster, h.
    zoster oticus, h.
herpesvirus (HV)
herpetic
    gingivitis, h.
    gingivostomatitis, h.

herpetic *(continued)*
    neuralgia, h.
    sore throat, h.
    stomatitis, h.
    tonsillitis, h.
herpetiform
herpetism
Hertwig sheath
hertz (Hz)
Heryng sign
Herzfeld ear forceps
Hess tonsil expressor
Hesselbach plexus
heterodont dentition
heterogeusia
heterologous
heterophonia
heterosmia
Heyman
    law, H.
    nasal forceps, H.
    nasal scissors, H.
Heyman-Paparella scissors
H-flu (Haemophilus influenzae)
HFS (hemifacial spasm)
HH (hiatal hernia)
hiatal
    esophagism, h.
    hernia, h. (HH)
    insufficiency, h.
hiation
hiatus
    esophageal h.
    facial canal, h. of
    fallopian canal, h. of
    maxillary h.
    maxillary sinus, h. of
    oesophageus, h.
    semilunaris, h.
hiatus hernia
Hibbs mouth gag
hiccough
hiccup
Hickman catheter
hidrotic ectodermal dysplasia
Hiebert esophageal suture spoon

high-frequency deafness
high-power magnification
high-speed drill
Highmore antrum
highmori
   sinus maxillaris, h.
highmoritis
Hilger
   facial nerve stimulator, H.
   mastoid obliteration procedure, H.
   tracheal tube, H.
Hill
   antireflux procedure, H.
   cluster harvest technique, H.
   posterior gastropexy, H.
Hi-Lo Jet tracheal tube
Hilsinger tonsillar knife
Hilton
   muscle, H.
   sac, H.
himantosis
Hinderer malar prosthesis
hinge
   axis, h.
   -axis point, h.
   bow, h.
   joint, h.
   movement, h.
hippocratic
   angina, h.
   face, h.
hircus
Hirschfeld canals
hirudiniasis
His
   canal, H.
   duct, H.
Hismanal
histamine
   cephalalgia, h.
   headache, h.
   receptor, h.
histaminic
histiocytoma
histiocytosis-X
histoplasmosis

histiocytosis
histrionic
   paralysis, h.
   spasm, h.
Hitzig test
HIV (human immunodeficiency virus)
hives
HMD (hyaline membrane disease)
hoarse
   voice, h.
hoarseness
hockey-stick
   incision, h.
   knife, h.
Hodgkin disease
hoe
   scaler, h.
Hoffman
   ear forceps, H.
   ear punch, H.
   ear rongeur, H.
Holdaway
   line, H.
   ratio, H.
Holinger
   applicator, H.
   bronchoscope, H.
   bronchoscopic magnet, H.
   bronchoscopie telescope, H.
   dissector, H.
   esophagoscope, H.
   hook-on folding laryngoscope, H.
   slotted laryngoscope, H.
Holinger-Garfield laryngoscope
Holinger-Jackson bronchoscope
Hollinger silver tracheotomy tube
Hollister laryngoscope
hollow
   Sebileau h.
Holmes
   gouge, H.
   nasopharyngoscope, H.
   otoplasty, H.
holoprosencephaly
Holz phlegmon
Holzheimer mastoid retractor

homeotransplantation
homodont dentition
homograft
homologous
homoplasty
Hong Kong ear
hood oxygen
hook
   muscle h.
   palate h.
hook-on
   bronchoscope, h.
   laryngoscope, h.
   loupe, h.
Hopkins 70 degree rigid telescope
Hopp
   anterior commissure laryngoscope blade, H.
   laryngoscope, H.
Hopp-Morrison laryngoscope
Hoppman polyp
horehound
Horgan procedure
horizontal
   canal, h.
   overlap, h.
   wedge lip resection, h.
hormion
Hormodendrum
hormonal gingivitis
Horn endo-otoprobe
horn of pulp
Horner
   syndrome, H.
   teeth, H.
horse asthma
horsehair suture
Horton
   arteritis, H.
   headache, H.
   syndrome, H.
hot
   cross bun skull, h.
   potato voice, h.
   weather ear, h.
hottentotism

Hotz
   ear applicator, H.
   ear curette, H.
Hough
   auger, H.
   crurotomy nipper, H.
   drum scraper, H.
   excavator hoe, H.
   footplate auger, H.
   footplate pick, H.
   hoe, H.
   oval-window excavator, H.
   spatula elevator, H.
   stapedectomy, H.
   stapedial footplate auger, H.
   tympanoplasty knife, H.
   whirlybird excavator, H.
Hough-Saunders stapes hoe
hour-glass anterior commissure laryngoscope
Hourin tonsil needle
House
   adaptor, H.
   alligator crimper forceps, H.
   alligator-strut forceps, H.
   chisel, H.
   crural hook, H.
   cup forceps, H.
   curette, H.
   drum elevator, H.
   elevator, H.
   endolymphatic shunt tube, H.
   footplate chisel, H.
   forceps, H.
   Gimmick stapes elevator, H.
   hook, H.
   incudostapedial joint knife, H.
   incus replacement prosthesis, H.
   irrigator, H.
   knife, H.
   needle, H.
   oiler tip, H.
   oval-window hook, H.
   piston, H.
   prosthesis, H.
   rod, H.

House *(continued)*
    scissors, H.
    separator, H.
    sickle knife, H.
    stapedectomy, H.
    tapping hammer, H.
    tube, H.
    tympanoplasty knife, H.
    wire, H.
    wire-fat prosthesis, H.
    wire stapes prosthesis, H.
House-Barbara needle
House-Dieter malleus nipper
House-Paparella stapes curette
House-Rosen needle
House-Urban
    gold ear marker, H.
    retractor, H.
House-Wullstein cup forceps
Howard tonsil-ligating forceps
Howarth operation
Hudson all-clear nasal cannula
Hueter maneuver
Hufford esophagoscope
Hu-Friedy dental bur
Hugier
    canal, H.
    sinus, H.
human immunodeficiency virus (HIV)
Humby knife
humid asthma
humidifier
humidity
Hunt
    disease, H.
    neuralgia, H.
Hunter glossitis
Hunter-Schreger bands
hunterian
Hupp tracheal retractor
Hurd
    elevator, H.
    forceps, H.
    reversible septal ridge forceps, H.
    tonsil dissector, H.
Hurd-Weder tonsil dissector

Hurler syndrome
Hurler-Scheie syndrome
Hurst
    esophageal bougie, H.
    mercury-filled dilator, H.
Hurthle cells
Hurwitz esophageal clamp
Huschke
    auditory teeth, H.
    canal, H.
    foramen, H.
    valve, H.
Husks mastoid rongeur
Hutchinson
    facies, H.
    incisors, H.
    teeth, H.
    triad, H.
HV (herpesvirus)
hyaline
    cartilage, h.
    membrane disease, h. (HMD)
hydrocephalus
    otitic h.
hydrocephaly
hydrocodone bitartrate
hydrocolloid
hydroconion
hydroglossa
hydroparotitis
hydrops
    labyrinthine h.
hydrorrhea
hydrotis
hydrotympanum
hydroxapatite
    cement, h.
    ossicular prosthesis, h.
Hyfrecator
hygiene
hygienist
hygroma
    colli, c.
    cystic h.
hygromatous
hygrostomia

Hynes pharyngoplasty
hyobasioglossus
hyobranchial cleft
hyoepiglottic
  folds, h.
  ligament, h.
hyoepiglottidean
hyoglossal
hyoglossus
hyoid
  arch, h.
  bar, h.
  bone, h.
  bursa, h.
  cleft, h.
hyomandibular cleft
hyopharyngeus
hyothyroid
  ligament, h.
  membrane, h.
hypacousia
hypacusia
hypacusis
hyparterial bronchus
hyperacuity
hyperacusis
hyperacute
hyperalgesia
hypercementosis
hyperdontia
hyperechema
hyperemia
hyperemic
hyperequilibrium
hyperesthesia
hypergasia
hypergeusia
hyperglandular
hyperkeratosis
  lacunaris, h.
hypermotility
hypernasal
hypernasality
hypernephroma
hyperorexia
hyperosmia

hyperosphresia
hyperostosis
  frontal internal h.
  infantile cortical h.
  Morgagni h.
hyperpallesthesia
hyperparathyroidism
hyperphonesis
hyperphonia
hyperpigmentation
hyperpigmented
hyperpituitarism
hyperplasia
  angiolymphoid h.
  cementum h.
  chronic perforating pulp h.
  Dilantin h.
  fibrous inflammatory h.
  gingival h.
hyperplastic
  gingivitis, h.
  gums, h.
hyperptyalism
hyperrhinoplasty
hypersalivation
hypersialosis
hypertaurodontism
hypertelorism
hyperthyroidism
hyperthyrosis
hypertrophic
  catarrh, h.
  tonsils, h.
hypertrophied
  tonsils, h.
hypertrophy
hyperventilation
hyperventilate
hypnodontia
hypnodontics
hypoacusis
hypobaropathy
hypobranchial eminence
hypocalcification
hypocalcipectic
hypocalcipexy

hypocone
hypoconid
hypoconulid
hypodontia
hypoergy
hypoesthesia
hypogeusia
   idiopathic h.
hypoglossal
   alternating hemiplegia, h.
   area, h.
   canal, h.
   nerve, h.
hypoglottis
hypognathous
hypognathus
hypohidrotic ectodermal dysplasia
hypolaryngeal
hypolarynx
hypomotility
hypomyxia
hyponasal
hyponasality
hypopallesthesia
hypoparathyreosis
hypoparathyroidism
hypopharyngeal
hypopharyngectomy
hypopharyngoscope
hypopharyngoscopy
hypopharyngeal
hypopharynx
hypophonia
hypophysial

hypophysial *(continued)*
   fossa, h.
hypophysis
hypophysitis
hypopituitarism
hypoplasia
   enamel h.
   focal dermal h.
   Turner h.
hypopnea
hypopneic
hyposalivation
hyposensitization
hyposialadenitis
hyposialosis
hyposmia
hyposphresia
hypostomia
hypotelorism
hypothyroid
hypothyroidism
hypotympanotomy
hypotympanum
hypoxia
hypsistaphylia
hypsistenocephalic
hypsodont
Hyrtl
   loop, H.
   recess, H.
hysterical
   deafness, h.
   vertigo, h.
Hz (hertz)

Additional entries

I

IA (internal auditory)
IAC (internal auditory canal)
IAM (internal auditory meatus)
iatrogenic
ichthyosis linguae
ICP (intracranial pressure)
icteric sputum
I&D (incision and drainage)
idioglossia
idioglottic
I/E ratio (inspiratory/expiratory ratio)
iliac crest bone graft
Iliff
    blepharochalasis forceps, I.
    technique, I.
illuminated nasal speculum
IM (infectious mononucleosis)
imbrication lines of Pickerill
immediate
    denture, i.
    -insertion denture, i.
immune
    response, i.
    system, i.
immunity
immunization
immunize
immunocompromised
immunodeficiency
immunodepression
immunohistochemistry
immunosuppressed
immunosuppression
immunotherapy
IMPA (incisal mandibular plane angle)
impacted
    cerumen, i.
    tooth, i.
impaction
impairment
impedance
    acoustic i.
Imperatori forceps

impetiginous cheilitis
impetigo
implant
    cochlear i.
    dental i.
    endodontic i.
    endosseous i.
    endosteal i.
    intraperiosteal i.
    magnet i.
    osseointegrated i.
    subperiosteal i.
    tooth i.
implant abutment
implant denture
implantation tooth
implanted tooth
implantodontics
implantodontist
implantodontology
implantologist
implantology
impression
    bridge i.
    cleft palate i.
    complete denture i.
    dental i.
    direct bone i.
    final i.
    lower i.
    mandibular i.
    maxillary i.
    partial denture i.
    preliminary i.
    primary i.
    secondary i.
    upper i.
impression area
impression materials
impression tray
impressive aphasia
IMV (intermittent mandatory ventilation)
incentive spirometry

index

in centric
incisal
    angle, i.
    canal, i.
    cavity, i.
    edge, i.
    guide angle, i.
    mandibular plane angle, i. (IMPA)
incision and drainage (I&D)
incisive
    bone, i.
    canal, i.
    duct, i.
incisolabial
incisolingual
incisoproximal
incisor
    central i.
    first i.
    Hutchinson i's
    lateral i.
    medial i.
    second i.
    shovel-shaped i's
    winged i.
incisor crest
incisor duct
incisor teeth
incisura (pl. incisurae)
incisurae (pl. of incisura)
incisure
    digastric i. of temporal bone
    ear, i. of
    ethmoidal i.
    interarytenoid i. of larynx
    jugular i.
    lacrimal i. of maxilla
    mandible, i. of
    mastoid i. of temporal bone
    maxillary i.
    nasal i.
    palatine i.
    palatine i. of Henle
    pterygoid i.
    Rivinus i.
    semilunar i. of mandible

incisure *(continued)*
    sigmoid i. of mandible
    sphenopalatine i. of palatine bone
    supraorbital i.
    thyroid i.
inclusion
    dental i.
incompetent
    esophageal sphincter, i.
    palatal syndrome, i.
incontentia
    pigmenti, i.
incostapedial
incremental lines
incrustation
incudal
incudectomy
incudiform
incudomalleal
incudomalleolar
    articulation, i.
    joint, i.
incudopexy
incudostapedial (IS)
    articulation, i.
    joint, i.
    joint knife, i.
    knife, i.
incudostapediopexy
incus
    bone, i.
    hook, i.
    replacement prosthesis, i.
    repositioning, i.
index
    alveolar i.
    auricular i.
    auriculoparietal i.
    auriculovertical i.
    basilar i.
    cephalic i.
    cranial i.
    dental i.
    DMF i. (decayed, missing, filled teeth)
    facial i.
    Flower i.

index *(continued)*
    gnathic i.
    maxilloalveolar i.
    nasal i.
    oral hygiene i.
    palatal i.
    palatine i.
    palatomaxillary i.
    periodontal i.
    Ramfjord i.
    short increment sensitivity i. (SISI)
    zygomaticoauricular i.
Indian
    flap, I.
    operation, I.
    rhinoplasty, I.
    rotation flap, I.
    skin flap operation, I.
indirect laryngoscopy
infant
    Ambu resuscitator, i.
    respiratory distress syndrome, i. (IRDS)
infection
    mediated, i.-
infectious
    asthmatic bronchitis, i.
    esophagitis, i.
    mononucleosis, i. (IM)
infectiousness
infective
    asthma, i.
infectivity
inferior
    carotid triangle, i.
    esophageal sphincter, i.
    laryngotomy, i.
    lingular bronchus, i.
    maxilla, i.
    nasal concha, i.
    pole of thyroid, i.
    tracheotomy, i.
    turbinate, i.
    turbinate firing, i.
inflamed
inflammation

influenza
    virus, i.
influenzal
infrabony pocket
infrabulge
infraclusion
infraconstrictor
infracture
infradentale
infraglottic cavity
infrahyoid bursa
inframandibular
inframaxillary
infraocclusion
infraorbital
    canal, i.
    foramen, i.
    nerve, i.
    pouching, i.
    rim, i.
infraoral
infraorbitomeatal line
infratemporal
    crest, i.
    fossa, i.
    surface of maxilla, i.
infratonsillar
infratubal
infraversion
infundibula (pl. of infundibulum)
infundibular
infundibuliform
infundibulum (pl. infundibula)
    ethmoidal i.
    nose, i. of
Ingals speculum
Ingersoll
    adenoid curette, I.
    tonsil needle, I.
ingest
ingested
ingestion
Ingrassia apophyses
inhalant
    antigens, i.
inhalation

inhalation *(continued)*
    bronchography, i.
    therapy, i.
inhale
inhaler
iniac
iniad
inial
inion
initial apnea
injected
    eardrum, i.
    pharynx, i.
    tonsils, i.
    tympanic membrane, i.
injection
inlay
    casting wax, i.
    bone graft, i.
    pattern wax, i.
inner ear
    deafness, i.
innervate
innervation
inorganic dust
insalivation
insane ear
insert
    intramucosal i.
    mucosal i.
inspirate
inspiration
inspirator
inspiratory
    spasm, i.
    stridor, i.
inspiratory/expiratory ratio (I/E ratio)
inspire
InspirEase
inspirometer
Inspiron Accur Ox Mask
inspissated
    cerumen, i.
inspissation
inspissator
instill
instillation
intake and output (I&O)
Intal
intellectual aphasia
interalveolar
interarch
interarytenoid
    muscle, i.
    notch, i.
intercanalicular
intercartilaginous
    incision, i.
    ossification, i.
intercavernous
    sinuses, i.
interclinoid
intercricothyrotomy
intercristal
intercurrent
intercuspation
intercusping
interdental
    canals, i.
    cells, i.
    cleft, i.
    gingiva, i.
interdentale
interdentium
interfacial
    canals, i.
interference
interferometer
interferometry
interfollicular cells
interfrontal
interfurca (pl. interfurcae)
interfurcae (pl. of interfurca)
intergemmal
interglobular
    dentin, i.
    spaces, i.
intergonial
interim denture
interjectional speech
interlabial
intermaxillary

intermaxillary *(continued)*
  anchorage, i.
  elastics, i.
  fixation, i.
  wiring, i.
intermediate abutment
intermittent mandatory ventilation (IMV)
internal
  acoustic meatus, i.
  auditory, i. (IA)
  auditory canal, i. (IAC)
  auditory meatus, i. (IAM)
  caries, i.
  ear, i.
  nose, n.
  pharyngotomy, i.
internarial
internasal
interocclusal
interorbital
interosseous
  wire fixation, i.
interparietal
INTERPLAK home plaque removal instrument
interpolate
interpolation
Interpore-200
interpose
interposition
  arthroplasty, i.
interpositional
  implant, i.
interproximal
  gingiva, i.
  radiography, i.
interradicular alveoplasty
interridge
interseptal alveoplasty
interstitial gingivitis
intertragic
  notch, i.
intertrigo
  labialis, i.
intertubular dentin
in toto

intra-aural
intrabronchial
intrabuccal
intracanalicular
intracapsular temporomandibular joint arthroplasty
intracranial pressure (ICP)
intragemmal
intraglandular
intrahyoid
intralaryngeal
intralingual
intramastoid
  abscess, i.
intramastoiditis
intramural
intranarial
intranasal
  antrum, i.
  antrum speculum, i.
  balloon, i.
  block, i.
  bone lever, i.
  ethmoidectomy, i.
  hammer, i.
  intercartilaginous incision, i.
  packing, i.
  punch, i.
  saw, i.
  sinusotomy, i.
  splint, i.
  tube, i.
intraoral
  anchorage, i.
  wire, i.
intraorbital
intraparietal
intraperiosteal implant
intrapulpal
intraseptal alveoplasty
intrathyroid
  cartilage, i.
intratonsillar
intratracheal
intrinsic asthma
intubation

intubation *(continued)*
   anesthesia, i.
   laryngoscope, i.
intratympanic
intrinsic
   asthma, i.
   laryngeal muscle, i.
   lingual muscle, i.
   tongue muscle branch, i.
introitus oesophagi
intubate
intubation
   endotracheal i.
   nasal i.
   nasoendotracheal i.
   nasogastric i.
   nasotracheal i.
   oral i.
   orotracheal i.
intubator
intumescentia tympanica
investing
   pattern, i. the
   tissue, i.
   vacuum i.
investment
   cast, i.
inviscation
involucrum
I&O (intake and output)
iodide goiter
iodine mumps
iodoform gauze
ipecac
ipsilateral
Ipsoclip
IRDS (infant respiratory distress syndrome)
irradiate
irradiated rib cartilage
irradiation
irrigate
irrigator
IS (incudostapedial)
islands of Calleja

isocyanate asthma
isodontic
isograft
isolated abutment
Israel
   Benzedrine vaporizer, I.
   nasal rasp, I.
   tonsillar dissector, I.
isthmectomy
isthmi (pl. of isthmus)
isthmic
isthmitis
isthmoparalysis
isthmoplegia
isthmospasm
isthmus (pl. isthmi)
   auditory tube, i. of
   cartilage of auricle, i. of
   eustachian tube, i. of
   fauces, i. of
   faucium, i.
   glandulae thyroideae, i.
   oropharyngeal i.
   pharyngeal i.
   pharyngonasal i.
   pharyngo-oral i.
   thyroid gland, i. of
   tubae auditivae, i.
Italian
   flap, I.
   operation, I.
Itard-Cholewa sign
ITE (in the ear) hearing aid
iter
   chordae, i.
iteral
Ivan laryngeal applicator
Iverson dermabrader
Ivor Lewis
   esophagectomy, I.
   esophagogastrectomy, I.
ivory of teeth
Ivy
   loop wiring, I.
   mastoid rongeur, I.

J

jacket
  Minerva j.
  porcelain j.
jacket crown
jackscrew
Jackson
  appliance, J.
  atomizer, J.
  bougie, J.
  bronchoscope, J.
  crib, J.
  esophageal bougie, J.
  esophagoscope, J.
  forceps, J.
  full-lumen esophagoscope, J.
  goiter retractor, J.
  laryngeal applicator, J.
  laryngofissure forceps, J.
  laryngoscope, J.
  laryngostat, J.
  safety triangle, J.
  scissors, J.
  sign, J.
  sliding laryngoscope, J.
  syndrome, J.
  tracheal hook, J.
  tracheoscope, J.
  tracheotomic bistoury, J.
jacksonian
  seizure, j.
Jacobson
  anastomosis, J.
  canal, J.
  cartilage, J.
  goiter retractor, J.
  nerve, J.
  organ, J.
  sulcus, J.
Jacquart angle
Jadelot lines
Jako
  facial nerve monitor, J.
  laryngeal microinstruments, J.

Jako *(continued)*
  laryngeal microscissors, J.
  laryngoscope, J.
  microlaryngeal grasping forceps, J.
  suspension otoscope, J.
Jako-Pilling
  knot pusher, J.
  laryngoscope, J.
Jalaguier cleft lip procedure
Jameson caliper
Janetta procedure
Jansen
  bayonet nasal forceps, J.
  ear forceps, J.
  mastoid raspatory, J.
  mastoid rongeur, J.
  mouth gag, J.
  operation, J.
  retractor, J.
Jansen-Gifford mastoid retractor
Jansen-Horgan procedure
Jansen-Middleton
  nasal-cutting forceps, J.
  septotomy forceps, J.
  septum-cutting forceps, J.
Jansen-Newhart mastoid probe
Jansen-Struycken septal forceps
Jansen-Wagner mastoid retractor
jargon aphasia
Jarvis
  operation, J.
  snare, J.
Jasbee esophagoscope
Javid shunt
jaw
  bird-beak j.
  cleft j.
  crackling j.
  Hapsburg j.
  lower j.
  parrot j.
  phossy j.
  pipe j.

jaw *(continued)*
   upper j.
jaw bone
jaw jerk
jaw joint
jaw-neck resection
jaw relation record
jaw repositioning
jaw thrust maneuver
jaw-winking syndrome
Jazbi
   nasal instrument set, J.
   suction tonsillar dissector, J.
Jefferson fracture
Jelenko arch bars
Jennings mouth gag
Jennings Loktite mouth gag
Jennings-Skillern mouth gag
Jerger tympanogram (type A/B/C)
jerk nystagmus
Jesberg
   bronchoscope, J.
   clamp, J.
   esophagoscope, J.
   infant bronchoscope, J.
jet
   humidifier, j.
   nebulizer, j.
   spray, j.
Jewitt classification
Johnson
   esophagogastrostomy, J.
   method, J.
   tonsillar punch, J.
   twin-wire appliance, J.
Johnson-Stevens disease
Jones
   curette, J.
   lacrimal canaliculus dilator, J.
   nasal splint, J.
Jonnson maneuver
Jordan
   stapedectomy knife, J.
   strut-measuring instrument, J.
Jordan-Day
   bur, J.

Jordan-Day *(continued)*
   drill, J.
Joseph
   clamp, J.
   elevator, J.
   knife, J.
   otoplasty, J.
   periosteotome, J.
   rhinoplasty, J.
   scissors, J.
   septal bar, J.
   septal fracture appliance, J.
   serrated scissors, J.
Joseph-Maltz nasal saw
jowl
Juers ear curette
Juers-Lempert forceps
juga (pl. of jugum)
jugal
   bone, j.
   process, j.
   suture, j.
jugale
jugate
jugulodigastric
jugomaxillary
jugular
   arch, j.
   eminence, j.
   floor, j.
   foramen, j.
   fossa, j.
   ganglion, j.
   process, j.
   vein, j.
   venous distention, j. (JVD)
   wall, j.
jugulodiastric
   lymph nodes, j.
jugum (pl. juga)
   petrosum, j.
   sphenoidale, j.
Juhn tympanocentesis trap
jumbled speech
jump
   flap, j.

jump *(continued)*
    graft, j.
jumping the bite
    appliance, j.
junction
    amelodentinal j.
    cardioesophageal j.
    cementodentinal j.
    cementoenamel j.
    dentinocemental j.
    dentinoenamel j.
    dentogingival j.
    esophagogastric j. (EGJ)
    gastroesophageal j.

junction *(continued)*
    mucocutaneous j.
    mucogingival j.
junctional epithelium
junctura (pl. juncturae)
juncturae (pl. of junctura)
June cold
Jung muscle
Jurasz laryngeal forceps
Juri scalp flap
jutting
    jaw, j.
    mandible, j.
JVD (jugular venous distention)

Additional entries

K

Kahler
    bronchoscopic forceps, K.
    laryngeal biopsy forceps, K.
Kanner syndrome
kaolin
Karamar-Mailatt tarsorrhaphy clamp
karaya
    adhesive, k.
    gum, k.
Karfik classification
Karroo syndrome
Kartagener syndrome
Kawasaki disease
Kaye technique
Kazanjian
    button, K.
    forceps, K.
    nasal-cutting forceps, K.
    nasal hump-cutting forceps, K.
    operation, K.
    scissors, K.
    shears, K.
    splint, K.
    T-bar, K.
Kearns-Sayre syndrome
Keegan operation
Keen point
Kehrer reflex
Keith needle
Kelly
    adenotome, K.
    clamp, K.
    operation, K.
keloid
    acne k.
    gums, k. of
Kennedy
    bar, K.
    classification, K.
Kent metallic condyle
Keofeed feeding tube
keratinize
kerato cyst

keratosis
    linguae, k.
    obturans, k.
    pharyngea, k.
Kerlix
Kernig sign
Kerrison mastoid rongeur
Kerrison-Costen ear rongeur
Kesling
    appliance, K.
    spring, K.
Kestenbaum operation
key-and-keyway attachment
Khodadad microclip forceps
kHz (kilohertz)
Kiel graft
Kiesselbach
    area, K.
    plexus, K.
killed-measles vaccine (MKV)
Killian
    antrum cannula, K.
    bronchoscope, K.
    chisel, K.
    elevator, K.
    frontal sinusotomy procedure, K.
    knife, K.
    nasal speculum, K.
    operation, K.
    tonsil knife, K.
    washing tube, K.
Killian-Freer operation
Killian-King goiter retractor
Killian-Lynch laryngoscope
Kilner
    cleft lip procedure, K.
    mouth gag, K.
Kilner-Dott mouth gag
Kilner-Doughty mouth gag
Kilner-Lynch laryngoscope
Kilner-McLarren procedure
kilohertz (kHz)
kinematic face-bow

King
    goiter retractor, K.
    vocal cord operation, K.
King-Hurd tonsil dissectomy
Kingsley
    appliance, K.
    plate, K.
    splint, K.
kiotome
kiotomy
Kirchner diverticulum
Kirkland knife
Kirkpatrick tonsil forceps
Kirschner
    diverticulum, K.
    wire, K.
Kirstein method
Kisch reflex
kissing tonsils
Kistner
    tracheal button, K.
    tracheostomy tube, K.
Kitlowski otoplasty
Kitner thyroid-packing forceps
Klaff septal speculum
Klebsiella
    rhinoscleromatis, K.
Kleenspec
    disposable laryngoscope, K.
    otoscope adapter, K.
Kleinsasser
    anterior commissure laryngoscope, K.
    laryngeal microsurgery instruments, K.
    microlaryngeal forceps, K.
    operating laryngoscope, K.
    ratcheted needle-holder, K.
Klemme gasserian ganglion retractor
Klestadt cyst
Klumpke paralysis
Knapp
    forceps, K.
    scissors, K.
Knapt scissors
knife
    gold k.

knife *(continued)*
    interdental k.
    periodontal k.
    plaster k.
Knight
    nasal forceps, K.
    scissors, K.
    turbinate forceps, K.
Knight-Sluder forceps
Knoop hardness test
Koch director
Kocher
    clamp, K.
    collar incision, K.
    operation, K.
Koffler forceps
Koffler-Lillie forceps
Kolle-Lexer otoplasty
Kolliker membrane
Konig
    graft, K.
    rods, K.
kophemia
Koplik spots
Kopp asthma
Korff fibers
Korner meatoplasty
koronion
Korte-Ballance operation
Kos cannula
Kostecka technique for mandibular prognathism
Kowalzig procedure
Koyter muscle
Krabbe disease
Kramer ear speculum
Krause
    cannula, K.
    ear knife, K.
    ear snare, K.
    forceps, K.
    glands, K.
    membrane, K.
    nasal snare, K.
    operation, K.
Krause-Wolfe graft

Kretschmann space
Krimer operation
Kronlein operation
K/S-Allis forceps
Kuhnt operation
Kussmaul
  aphasia, K.
  respiration, K.
Kuster operation

Kuttner
  parotid repair, K.
  ganglion, K.
Kwapis instrument
Kyle
  crypt knife, K.
  ear applicator, K.
  nasal speculum, K.

Additional entries

L

L (lingual)
LA (linguoaxial)
LAA (labioaxial)
LAAG (labioaxiogingival)
labia (pl. of labium)
   oris, l.
labial
   angles, l.
   bar, l.
   cavity, l.
   curve, l.
   gingiva, l.
   tooth, l.
labialism
labially
labioalveolar
labioaxial (LAA)
labioaxiogingival (LAAG)
labiocervical (LAC)
labiochorea
labioclination
labiodental
   lamina, l.
labiogingival (LAG)
labioglossolaryngeal
labioglossopharyngeal
labiograph
labioincisal (LAI)
labiolingual (LAL)
   appliance, l.
   diameter, l.
labiologic
labiology
labiomental
labiomycosis
labionasal
labiopalatine
labioplacement
labioplasty
labiotenaculum
labioversion
labium (pl. labia)
   mandibulare, l.

labium (pl. labia) *(continued)*
   maxillare, l.
   oris, l.
   tympanicum, l.
   vestibulare, l.
   vocale, l.
Laborde
   method, L.
   tracheal dilator, L.
labrale
   inferius, l.
   superius, l.
labyrinth
   acoustic l.
   bony l.
   cochlear l.
   cortical l.
   endolymphatic l.
   ethmoid, l. of
   ethmoidal l.
   Ludwig l.
   membranous l.
   nonacoustic l.
   olfactory l.
   osseous l.
   perilymphatic l.
   statokinetic l.
   vestibular l.
labyrinth vestibule
labyrinthectomy
labyrinthi (pl. of labyrinthus)
labyrinthic
   ataxia, l.
labyrinthine
   deafness, l.
   hydrops, l.
   nystagmus, l.
   torticollis, l.
   vertigo, l.
labyrinthitis
   circumscribed l.
labyrinthodont
labyrinthosis

labyrinthotomy
labyrinthus (pl. labyrinthi)
   cochlearis, l.
   ethmoidalis, l.
   membranaceus, l.
   osseus, l.
   vestibularis, l.
LAC (labiocervical)
lacrimal
   abscess, l.
   apparatus, l.
   bone, l.
   calculus, l.
   crest, l.
   duct, l.
   fold, l.
   gland, l.
   lake, l.
   punctum, l.
   reflex, l.
   sac, l.
lacrimation
lacrimator
lacrimatory
lacrimo-auriculo-dento-digital syndrome
lacrimoconchal
lacrimoethmoidal
lacrimomaxillary
lacrimonasal
   duct, l.
lacrimotome
lacrimotomy
lacrimoturbinal
lactated Ringer's solution
lacuna (pl. lacunae)
lacunae (pl. of lacuna)
lacunar
   angina, l.
   tonsillitis, l.
Laennec catarrh
Laforce
   adenotome, L.
   hemostatic tonsillectome, L.
   knife spud, L.
   tonsillectomy, L.
Laforce-Grieshaber adenotome

Laforce Stevenson adenotome
LAG (labiogingival or linguoaxiogingival)
lagena
lageniform
Lagleyze eyelid technique
lagophthalmos
Lahey thyroid traction vulsellum forceps
LAI (labioincisal)
Laimer-Haeckerman area
LAL (labiolingual)
laliatry
lallation
lalognosis
lalopathology
lalophobia
laloplegia
lalorrhea
Lalouette pyramid
lambdacism
lamella (pl. lamellae)
   enamel l.
lamellae (pl. of lamella)
lamellated
lamina (pl. laminae)
   alar l.
   basilar l.
   cribriform l.
   dental l.
   dentogingival l.
   dura, l.
   labiodental l.
   labiogingival l.
   labial l.
   palatine l. of maxilla
   papyracea, l.
   perpendicular l.
   pretracheal l.
   propria, l.
   pterygoid l.
   spiral l.
   vestibular l.
laminae (pl. of lamina)
laminated epithelium
Lamont
   elevator, L.

Lamont *(continued)*
   nasal rasp, L.
   nasal raspatory, L.
   nasal saw, L.
Lancaster technique
lance
lancet
   gingival l.
   gum l.
lancinating pain
landmark
   cephalometric l.
   craniometric l.
   orbital l.
Landolt operation
Landstrom muscle
Lane
   cleft palate needle, L.
   mouth gag, L.
Langdon Down disease
Lange
   antrum punch, L.
   mouth gag, L.
Langer lines
laniary
Lanz
   low-pressure cuff endotracheal tube, L.
   tracheostomy tube, L.
Larat treatment
LaRocca tube
Larsen syndrome
laryngalgia
laryngeal
   adhesion, l.
   aperture, l.
   applicator, l.
   atomizer, l.
   biopsy, l.
   biopsy forceps, l.
   block, l.
   cannula, l.
   cartilage, l.
   cavity, l.
   commissure, l.
   crisis, l.

laryngeal *(continued)*
   dilatation, l.
   dilator, l.
   diphtheria, l.
   dissector, l.
   diverticulum, l.
   drop operation, l.
   enterotome, l.
   forceps, l.
   intubation, l.
   keel, l.
   knife, l.
   lupus, l.
   mirror, l.
   nerve, l.
   nodule, l.
   paralysis, l.
   polyp, l.
   pouch, l.
   probe, l.
   prominence, l.
   prosthesis, l.
   punch, l.
   punch forceps, l.
   reconstruction, l.
   reflex, l.
   retractor, l.
   rotation forceps, l.
   saccule, l.
   saw, l.
   scissors, l.
   sinus, l.
   snare, l.
   spasm, l.
   speculum, l.
   sponging forceps, l.
   stenosis, l.
   stricture, l.
   stridor, l.
   swab, l.
   ventricle, l.
   vertigo, l.
   web, l.
laryngectomee
laryngectomize
laryngectomy

laryngectomy *(continued)*
  clamp, l.
  saw, l.
  tube, l.
laryngemphraxis
laryngendoscope
larynges (pl. of larynx)
laryngeus nerve
laryngismal
laryngismus
  paralyticus, l.
  stridulus, l.
laryngitic
laryngitis
  acute catarrhal l.
  atrophic l.
  chronic catarrhal l.
  croupous l.
  diphtheritic l.
  membranous l.
  phlegmonous l.
  sicca, l.
  stridulosa, l.
  subglottic l.
  syphilitic l.
  tuberculous l.
  vestibular l.
laryngocele
  ventricular l.
  ventricularis, l.
laryngocentesis
laryngoedema
laryngoesophagectomy
laryngofission
laryngofissure
  forceps, l.
  profilometer, l.
  retractor, l.
  saw, l.
  scissors, l.
  shears, l.
laryngogram
laryngograph
laryngography
  contrast l.
laryngohypopharynx

laryngologist
laryngology
laryngomalacia
laryngometry
laryngoparalysis
laryngopathy
laryngophantom
laryngopharyngeal
laryngopharyngectomy
laryngopharyngeus
laryngopharyngitis
laryngopharyngoesophagectomy
laryngopharyngography
laryngopharyngoscope
laryngopharyngeal
laryngopharynx
laryngophony
laryngophthisis
laryngoplasty
laryngoplegia
laryngoptosis
laryngopyocele
laryngorhinologist
laryngorhinology
laryngorrhagia
laryngorrhaphy
laryngorrhea
laryngoscleroma
laryngoscope
  battery handle, l.
  chest support holder, l.
  folding blade, l.
laryngoscopic
laryngoscopist
laryngoscopy
  direct l.
  indirect l.
  mirror l.
  suspension l.
laryngospasm
laryngostasis
laryngostat
  Jackson l.
laryngostenosis
  compression l.
  occlusion l.

laryngostomy
laryngostroboscope
laryngotome
laryngotomy
   complete l.
   inferior l.
   median l.
   subhyoid l.
   superior l.
   thyrohyoid l.
laryngotracheal
   reconstruction, l. (LTR)
   stenosis, l. (LTS)
laryngotracheitis
laryngotracheobronchitis (LTB)
laryngotracheobronchoscopy
laryngotracheoesophageal
   cleft, l.
laryngotracheoplasty
laryngotracheoscopy
laryngotracheotomy
laryngotyphoid
laryngovestibulitis
laryngoxerosis
larynx (pl. larynges)
   artificial l.
laser
late apnea
latellar
latent nystagmus
lateral
   caries, l.
   crural overlay technique, l.
   crus, l.
   nystagmus, l.
   pharyngotomy, l.
   process of malleus, l.
   recess of nasopharynx, l.
   wall, l.
laterality
lateralization
laterognathia
laterotrusion
Lathbury applicator
Latrobe retractor
LATS (long-acting thyroid stimulator)

laughing gas
Laumonier ganglion
Lauren operation
laws of articulation
Law view
layer
   adamantine l.
   ameloblastic l.
   circular l. of drumhead
   circular l. of tympanic membrane
   enamel l.
   granular l. of Tomes
   mucous l. of tympanic membrane
   odontoblastic l.
   palisade l.
   submantle l.
   subodontoblastic l.
   Tomes granular l.
   Weil basal l.
LC (linguocervical)
LD (linguodistal)
lead
   lines, l.
   stomatitis, l.
Leahey technique
leech therapy
leeching
Leake dacron mandible
Le Fort
   I, II, III fractures, L.
   apertognathia repair, L.
   maxillary reconstruction, L.
Legal disease
Leishmania
   braziliensis, L.
leishmaniasis
   American l.
   mucocutaneous l.
leishmanicidal
Lejeune
   applicator, L.
   scissors, L.
Leland knife
Lell
   esophagoscope, L.
   laryngofissure saw, L.

LeMesurier procedure
lemoparalysis
lemostenosis
Lempert
   bur, L.
   curette, L.
   elevator, L.
   fenestration, L.
   forceps, L.
   incision, L.
   knife, L.
   perforator, L.
   procedure, L.
   retractor, L.
Lempert-Colver speculum
Lennert classification
lenticular
   aphasia, l.
   knob, l.
   process of incus, l.
lentulo
Lentz tracheotomy tube
Lenz syndrome
leonine facies
leopard syndrome
Leo test
leprechaun facies
leptodontous
leptophonia
leptoprosopia
leptorrhine
leptostaphyline
Leredde syndrome
Lermoyez
   punch, L.
   syndrome, L.
LeRoy scalp clip applying forceps
LES (lower esophageal sphincter)
Lesch-Nyhan syndrine
Letterer-Siwe disease
Leudet tinnitus
leukemia
leukemic
leukodystrophy
leukoplakia
   buccalis, l.

leukoplakia *(continued)*
   lingualis, l.
   oral l.
   speckled l.
leukopoietic
levator
   anguli oris muscle, l.
   labii inferioris muscle, l.
   labii superioris alaeque nasi muscle, l.
   labii superioris muscle, l.
   menti muscle, l.
   musculi linguae, l.
   palati muscle, l.
   palpebrae superioris muscle, l.
   veli palatini muscle, l.
Lewin
   tonsil hemostat, L.
   tonsil screw, L.
Lewis
   loupe, L.
   mouth gag, L.
   nasal raspatory, L.
   rasp, L.
   scoop, L.
   snare, L.
   tongue depressor, L.
   tube, L.
   uvula retractor, L.
Lewy
   laryngoscope, L
   suspension, L.
   suspension apparatus, L.
Lexer
   lop ear technique, L.
   otoplasty, L.
LG (linguogingival)
LI (linguoincisal)
lichen planus
Lichtheim aphasia
Lichtwicz
   antral needle, L.
   trocar, L.
lid
   dermabrader, l.
   dermabrasion, l.
   -fracturing blepharoplasty, l.

lid *(continued)*
    lag, l.
    ptosis operation, l.
    -retracting hook, l.
    retractor, l.
    scalpel, l.
Liebenmann procedure
ligate
ligation
light reflex
ligneous thyroiditis
Lillie
    alligator scissors, L.
    antral trocar, L.
    attic cannula, L.
    attic hook, L.
    ear hook, L.
    frontal sinus probe, L.
    nasal speculum, L.
    sinus bone-nibbling rongeur, L.
    speculum, L.
    tonsillar scissors, L.
Lillie-Killian septal bone forceps
limbus
    alveolar l. of mandible
    alveolar l. of maxilla
    angulosus, l.
    lamina spiralis ossae, l.
    membranae tympani, l.
    palpebrales anteriores, l.
    palpebrales posteriores, l.
    sphenoidalis, l.
    spiral l.
limen (pl. limina)
    nasi, l.
limina (pl. of limen)
Lindeman-Silverstein tube
Lindholm
    anatomical tracheal tube, L.
    operating laryngoscope, L.
line
    accretion l's
    alveolobasilar l.
    alveolonasal l.
    auriculobregmatic l.
    base line

line *(continued)*
    basinasial l.
    basiobregmatic l.
    biauricular l.
    bismuth l.
    blue l.
    calcification l's
    Camper, l. of
    canthomeatal l.
    cervical l.
    Clapton l.
    copper l.
    Corrigan l.
    cricoclavicular l.
    De Salle l.
    developmental l's
    dynamic l's
    Ebner, l's of
    expression, l's of
    facial l.
    Fischgold bimastoid l.
    fulcrum l.
    genal l.
    gingival l.
    glabellomeatal l.
    Gottinger l.
    Granger l.
    gum l.
    imbrication l's of cementum
    incremental l's
    incremental l's of Retzius
    incremental l's of von Ebner
    infraorbitomeatal l.
    interauricular l.
    Jadelot l's
    labial l.
    lead l's
    lip l.
    mentomeatal l.
    mucogingival l.
    mylohyoid l.
    mylohyoidean l.
    nasobasal l.
    nasobasilar l.
    nasolabial l.
    nuchal l.

line *(continued)*
    oblique l. of mandible
    occlusion, l. of
    oculozygomatic l.
    Owen, l's of
    paraesophageal l.
    paratracheal l.
    Poirier l.
    precentral l.
    recessional l's
    Reid base l.
    relaxed skin tension l's
    Retzius, l. of
    Schoemaker l.
    Schreger, l's of
    sternomastoid l.
    supraorbital l.
    survey l.
    sylvian l.
    Thompson l.
    thyroid red l.
    Topinard l.
    Virchow l.
    white l. of pharynx
    Z l. of esophagus
line angle
liner
    cavity l.
    soft l.
lingoscope
lingua (pl. linguae)
    dissecta, l.
    frenata, l.
    geographica, l.
    nigra, l.
    plicata, l.
    villosa nigra, l.
linguae (pl. of lingua)
lingual (L)
    angles, l.
    aponeurosis, l.
    arch. l.
    bar, l.
    block, l.
    cavity, l.
    duct, l.

lingual (L) *(continued)*
    flange, l.
    frenotomy, l.
    gingiva, l.
    glands, l.
    goiter, l.
    gyrus, l.
    hemorrhoid, l.
    inclination, l.
    lamina, l.
    lymph node, l.
    nerve, l.
    occlusion, l.
    papillae, l.
    quinsy, l.
    splint, l.
    surface of tooth, l.
    thyroid, l.
    tongue flap, l.
    tonsil, l.
    tonsillectome, l.
    tonsillectomy, l.
    thyroid, l.
    titubation, l.
    tongue flap, l.
    tonsil, l.
    tonsillitis, l.
linguale
lingualis
lingually
linguiform
lingula (pl. lingulae)
    lower jaw, l. of
    mandibular l.
    mandible, l. of
    sphenoid, l. of
    sphenoidal l.
lingulae (pl. of lingula)
lingular
lingulectomy
linguoaxial (LA)
linguoaxiogingival (LAG)
linguocervical (LC)
linguoclasia
linguoclination
linguoclusion

linguodental
linguodistal (LD)
linguofacial trunk
linguogingival (LG)
linguoincisal (LI)
linguomesial (LM)
linguo-occlusal (LO)
linguopapillitis
linguoplacement
linguopulpal
linguoversion
lion's teeth
lip
    articular l.
    cleft l.
    double l.
    Hapsburg l.
    inferior l.
    lower l.
    oral l's
    tympanic l.
    upper l.
    vestibule l.
lip adhesion procedure
lip biting
lip graft
lip pursing
lip reading
lip shave
lip sucking
lip switch flap
lipectomy
lipoma
lipomatous
lipostomy
Lipsett tip technique
liquefaction
liquefy
liquefying
    expectorant, l.
liquor
lisp
lisping
listing seagull incision
Liston operation
lithemic vertigo

Littauer
    ear-dressing forceps, L.
    nasal-dressing forceps, L.
    procedure, L.
Little area
Lizars operation
Lloyd esophagoscopic catheter
LM (linguomesial)
LO (linguo-occlusal)
loading dose
lobe
lobulated tongue
lobule
lobuli (pl. of lobulus)
lobulus (pl. lobuli)
localization audiometry
lockjaw
Lockwood ligament
Loebker tongue forceps
Logan bow
logokophosis
logopathia
logopedia
logopedics
logoplegia
logospasm
Lombard
    mastoid rongeur, L.
    test, L.
Lombard-Boies rongeur
long
    crus, l.
    process of incus, l.
    process of malleus, l.
    teeth, l.
lop ear
lophodont
Lorenz-Rees nasal rasp
Lorie
    antral trephine, L.
    tonsillar suture instrument, L.
Lothrop
    tonsillar knife, L.
    uvula retractor, L.
loupe
    magnification, l.

Love
    nasal splint, L.
    uvula retractor, L.
Lovelace thyroid traction vulsellum forceps
low tracheotomy
Low-Beer view
Lowenberg
    canal, L.
    forceps, L.
    scala, L.
lower
    esophageal sphincter, l. (LES)
    trapezius island musculocutaneous flap, l. (LTIMF)
Lowitt bodies
low-set ears
lozenge
L plate
LTB (laryngotracheobronchitis)
LTIMF (lower trapezius island musculocutaneous flap)
LTR (laryngotracheal reconstruction)
LTS (laryngotracheal stenosis)
L-type nose-bridge prosthesis
Luc operation
Lucae forceps
Luckett otoplasty
Ludwig
    angina, L.
    labyrinth, L.
    sinus applicator, L.
Luer
    tracheal cannula, L.
    tracheal double-ended retractor, L.
Luer-Whiting mastoid rongeur
lug
Luhr
    fixation system, L.
    mandibular plate, L.
    maxillofacial system, L.
    microplate, L.

Lukens tracheal double-ended retractor
Lukes-Collins classification
Lundy laryngoscope
lung bud
Luongo
    hand retractor, L.
    sphenoid irrigating cannula, L.
Luschka
    bursa, L.
    crypts, L.
    laryngeal cartilage, L.
    tonsil, L.
Lutz septal ridge-cutting forceps
Lutz-Splendore-Almeida disease
luxation
Lyme
    disease, L.
    titer, L.
lymph
    glands, l.
    sinus, l.
lymph node
    buccinator l.
    calcified l.
    facial l.
    infraorbital l.
    lingual l.
    mastoid l.
    maxillary l.
    neck, l. of
    paratracheal l.
    parotid l.
    preauricular l.
    retropharyngeal l.
    Rosenmuller l.
    shotty l.
    submaxillary l.
    submental l.
    supramandibular l.
    tongue, l. of
    tracheobronchial l.
lymphadenectasis

M

M (mesial)
Macewen triangle
MacFee neck flap
Machek technique
Machida
    bronchoscope, M.
    fiberoptic laryngoscope, M.
MacIntosh
    blade, M.
    laryngoscope, M.
Mack
    ear plugs, M.
    tonsillectome, M.
Mackenty
    antral tube, M.
    choanal plug, M.
    cleft palate knife, M.
    elevator, M.
    sphenoid punch, M.
    tube, M.
Mackenzie syndrome
Mackler esophageal tube
Maclay tonsillar scissors
macradenous
macroblepharia
macrocephalia
macrocheilia
macrocrania
macrodont
macrodontia
macrodontic
macrodontism
macrogenia
macrogingivae
macrogingival
macroglossia
    -ophthalmocele syndrome, m.
macrognathia
macrolabia
macroprosopia
macrorhinia
macrosmatic
macrostomia

macrotia
macrotooth
macula
    acoustic m.
    acusticae, m.
    acustica sacculi, m.
    communis, m.
    cribrosa, m.
    densa, m.
    flava laryngis, m.
    membranous labyrinth, m. of
    sacculi, m.
    utriculi, m.
macular
maculopapular rash
maculovesicular
MadaJet XL injector
Madelung neck
madreporic coral
magenta tongue
Magielski
    canal knife, M.
    chisel, M.
    needle, M.
    tonsil forceps, M.
Magill
    laryngoscope, M.
    tube, M.
Magna-Finder
Magnan movement
Magna-Site tissue expander
magnet implant
magnetic implant
magnification
    loupe m.
magnifying loupe
Magnum Oto-Tool system
Magnus technique
Mahoney intranasal antral speculum, M.
Mahorner thyroid retractor
Maier sinus
mainstem bronchus
mainstream aerosol

maintainer
   space m.
mal
   perforant palatin, m.
mala
malacotic teeth
malalignment
malalinement
malar
   arch, m.
   augmentation, m.
   bone, m.
   crest, m.
   elevator, m.
   eminence, m.
   flush, m.
   fracture, m.
   incision, m.
   lymph node, m.
   process of maxilla, m.
   prosthesis, m.
malarial deafness
malaris
Malassez rest
Malbran technique
maleruption
malformation
malformed
Malgaigne
   fossa, M.
   triangle, M.
Maliniac
   nasal raspatory, M.
   nasal retractor, M.
malinterdigitation
malleability
malleable
malleoincudal
   joint, m.
malleolar
malleotomy
mallet
malleus
   cutter, m.
   forceps, m.
   handle, m.

malleus *(continued)*
   nipper, m.
   punch, m.
Mallinckrodt Laser-Flex tube
Mallory-Weiss
   syndrome, M.
   tear, M.
maloccluded
malocclusal
malocclusion
   closed-bite m.
   open-bite m.
malomaxillary
Maloney
   bougie, M.
   dilator, M.
   endo-otoprobe, M.
   mercury-filled esophageal dilator, M.
malposed tooth
Maltz
   angle knife, M.
   bayonet saw, M.
   nasal saw, M.
   rasp, M.
Maltz-Anderson nasal rasp
Maltz-Lipsett nasal rasp
Manashil sialography catheter
Manchester cleft lip repair
Mandelbaum ear knife
mandible
   splint, m.
mandibula (pl. mandibulae)
mandibulae (pl. of mandibula)
mandibular
   advancement, m.
   angle, m.
   arch, m.
   arch bar, m.
   articulation, m.
   axis, m.
   block, m.
   canal, m.
   cartilage, m.
   cuspid, m.
   dentitional odontectomy, m.
   foramen, m.

mandibular *(continued)*
    fossa, m.
    gingiva, m.
    glide, m.
    horizontal deficiency, m.
    immobilization, m.
    lymph node, m.
    mobilization, m.
    nerve, m.
    notch, m.
    plane, m.
    port, m.
    prognathism, m.
    prosthesis, m.
    protraction, m.
    ramus, m.
    recontouring alveolectomy, m.
    reflex, m.
    ridge, m.
    setback, m.
    symphysis, m.
    torus, m.
mandibularis
mandibulectomy
mandibulofacial
    dysmorphia, m.
    dysostosis, m.
mandibulopharyngeal
mandibulosacral dysplasia
mandibulotomy
Mandl paint
mandrel
manometer
manometry
mantle
    dentin, m.
manubrium
    mallei, m.
    malleus, m. of
mappy tongue
Marax bronchodilator
marble bone disease
Marcks procedure
margin
    alveolar m.
    free gingival m.

margin *(continued)*
    free gum m.
    gingival m.
    gum m.
    infraorbital m. of maxilla
    lacrimal m. of maxilla
    malar m.
    mandible, m. of
    mastoid m.
    orbital m.
    parietal m.
    parietofrontal m.
    sphenoidal m.
    sphenotemporal m.
    squamous m.
    supraorbital m.
    tongue, m. of
    zygomatic m.
marginal
    gingiva, m.
    gingivitis, m.
    periodontitis, m.
marginoplasty
margo
    gingivalis, m.
    incisalis, m.
    infraorbitalis, m.
    lacrimalis, m.
    lateralis, m.
    linguae, l.
    mastoideus, m.
    nasalis, m.
    nasi, m.
    orbitalis, m.
    palpebrae, m.
    parietalis, m.
    sphenoidalis, m.
    supraorbitalis, m.
    zygomaticus, m.
Marie disease
Mark IV nasogastric tube
marking pencil
Maroon lip curette
marrow graft
Marsh Robinson procedure
Marshik

Marshik *(continued)*
    tonsillar forceps, M.
    tonsil-seizing forceps, M.
marsupialization
marsupialize
Martin
    hook, M.
    laryngectomy tube, M.
    lip retractor, M.
    nasopharyngeal biopsy forceps, M.
    palate elevator, M.
    throat scissors, M.
mask
masseter
masseteric
master cast
mastic
masticate
masticating surface
mastication
masticator abscess
masticatory
    apparatus, m.
    diplegia, m.
    force, m.
    habit, m.
mastiche
mastoid
    abscess, m.
    air cells, m.
    angle, m.
    antrotomy, m.
    antrum, m.
    bone, m.
    bowl, m.
    bur, m.
    canaliculus, m.
    catheter, m.
    cavity, m.
    cells, m.
    chisel, m.
    curette, m.
    dressing, m.
    emissary vein, m.
    fontanelle, m.
    foramen, m.

mastoid *(continued)*
    fossa, m.
    gouge, m.
    lymph nodes, m.
    mallet, m.
    notch, m.
    obliteration, m.
    packer, m.
    probe, m.
    process, m.
    raspatory, m.
    -retaining retractor, m.
    rongeur, m.
    rongeur forceps, m.
    scoop, m.
    search, m.
    searcher, m.
    sinus, m.
    suction tube, m.
    suture, m.
    tegmen, m.
    tip, m.
    wall, m.
mastoidal
mastoidale
mastoidalgia
mastoidea
mastoidectomy
    radical m.
    simple m.
mastoideocentesis
mastoideum
mastoiditis
    Bezold m.
    catarrhal m.
    coalescent m.
    externa, m.
    interna, m.
    sclerosing m.
    sclerotic m.
    silent m.
    suppurative m.
mastoidotomy
mastoidotympanectomy
masto-occipital
mastoparietal

mastosquamous
mat
  foil, m.
  gold, m.
materia
  alba, m.
  dentica, m.
material
  amalgam m.
  base m.
  baseplate m.
  dental m.
  impression m.
Mathieu tongue-seizing forceps
matrices (pl. of matrix)
matrix (pl. matrices)
  amalgam m.
matrix band
matrix retainer
matted node
mattress sutures
Maunder oral screw gag
maxilla (pl. maxillae)
maxillae (pl. of maxilla)
maxillary
  alveolectomy, m.
  alveoplasty, m.
  anchorage, m.
  angle, m.
  antrotomy, m.
  antrum, m.
  arch, m.
  articulation, m.
  canal, m.
  crest, m.
  cuspid, m.
  dental prosthesis, m.
  gingiva, m.
  lymph nodes, m.
  nerve, m.
  process, m.
  protraction, m.
  recontouring alveolectomy, m.
  ridge, m.
  sinus, m.
  sinusitis, m.

maxillary *(continued)*
  sinusotomy, m.
  spine, m.
  teeth, m.
  torus, m.
  tuberosity, m.
maxillectomy
maxillitis
maxillodental
maxilloethmoidectomy
maxillofacial
  appliance, m.
  prosthesis, m.
  surgery, m.
maxillojugal
maxillolabial
maxillomandibular
  anchorage, m.
  traction, m.
maxillopalatine
maxillopharyngeal
maxillotomy
Maxi-Myst vaporizer
Mayer
  nasal splint, M.
  position, M.
  view, M.
Mayo
  sign, M.
  stand, M.
MB (mesiobuccal)
MBO (mesiobucco-occlusal)
MBP (mesiobuccopulpal)
MC (mesiocervical)
McCabe
  canal knife, M.
  crurotomy saw, M.
  facial nerve dissection, M.
  flap knife dissector, M.
  rasp, M.
McCall festoon
McCarthy reflex
McCash-Randall procedure
McCaskey curette
McCoy septal forceps
McCurdy staphylorrhaphy needle

McDowell
    mouth gag, M.
    procedure, M.
McGee
    piston prosthesis, M.
    procedure, M.
McGhan facial implant
McGhan Micro-Torque hand engine
McGregor forehead flap
McHenry tonsillar artery forceps
McHugh
    facial nerve knife, M.
    flap knife, M.
    speculum, M.
McIvor mouth gag
McKay ear forceps
McKenzie sphenoid punch
McKesson
    mouth gag, M.
    mouth probe, M.
McNaught keel laryngeal prosthesis
McNeill-Goldmann blepharostat ring
McQuigg-Mixter bronchial forceps
McWhinnie dissector
McWhorter tonsillar forceps
MD (mesiodistal)
Mead
    lancet, M.
    mallet, M.
    mastoid rongeur, M.
measles
    atypical m.
    black m.
    German m.
    hemorrhagic m.
    three-day m.
meatal
    cartilage, m.
    flap, m.
meati (pl. of meatus)
meatoantrostomy
meatoantrotomy
meatoplasty
meatus (pl. meati)
    acoustic m.
    acusticus externus, m.

meatus (pl. meati) *(continued)*
    acusticus internus, m.
    auditorius, m.
    auditory m.
    conchae, m.
    external acoustic m.
    external auditory m.
    internal acoustic m.
    internal auditory m.
    nasal m.
    nasi communis, m.
    nasi inferior, m.
    nasi medius, m.
    nasi superior, m.
    nasopharyngeal m.
    nasopharyngeus, m.
    nose, m. of
mechanic bronchitis
mechanical
    condenser, m.
    cough, m.
    vertigo, m.
mechanism
    deglutition m.
    swallowing m.
Meckel
    cartilage, M.
    ganglion, M.
    plane, M.
    rod, M.
meckelectomy
median
    laryngotomy, m.
    rhomboid glossitis, m.
mediastinoscope
mediastinoscopy
mediator
medicinal leeches
Medicon-Jackson laryngeal forceps
medication-effect
Meding
    tonsil enucleator, M.
    tonsil enucleator tonometer, M.
Med-Neb respirator
Medrol Dosepak
megadont

megadontia
megaesophagus
megalodontia
megaloesophagus
megaloglossia
Meglin point
meiolabial flap
melanoglossia
melanoma
melanoplakia
melanoptysis
melanotrichia
   linguae, m.
melitoptyalism
melitoptyalon
Melkersson syndrome
Melkersson-Rosenthal syndrome
Meller operation
meloncus
melonoplasty
meloplasty
meloschisis
melotia
Melotte metal
Meltzer
   nasopharyngoscope, M.
   punch, M.
membrana (pl. membranae)
   basilaris ductus cochlearis, m.
   elastica laryngis, m.
   fibroelastica laryngis, m.
   mucosa nasi, m.
   spiralis ductus cochlearis, m.
   stapedis, m.
   tympani, m.
membranaceous
membranae (pl. of membrana)
membrane
   adamantine m.
   alveodental m.
   basilar m. of cochlear duct
   Brunn m.
   bucconasal m.
   buccopharyngeal m.
   Corti, m. of
   cricothyroid m.

membrane *(continued)*
   cricovocal m.
   croupous m.
   Debove m.
   dentinoenamel m.
   diphtheritic m.
   drum m.
   enamel m.
   endoral m.
   false m.
   fibroelastic m. of larynx
   Hannover intermediate m.
   hyoglossal m.
   hyothyroid m.
   Kolliker m.
   Krause m.
   laryngeal mucous m.
   lingual mucous m.
   mucous m.
   nasal mucous m.
   Nasmyth m.
   obturator m. of larynx
   olfactory m.
   oral m.
   oronasal m.
   oropharyngeal m.
   otolithic m.
   palatal mucous m.
   palatine m.
   paroral m.
   peridental m.
   periodontal m.
   pharyngeal m.
   pharyngeal mucous m.
   pharyngobasilar m.
   pituitary m. of nose
   Reissner m.
   Rivinus m.
   Scarpa m.
   schneiderian m.
   Shrapnell m.
   spiral m. of cochlear duct
   stapedial m.
   submucous m.
   tectorial m.
   thyreohyoid m.

membrane *(continued)*
    thyrohyoid m.
    tympanic m.
    vestibular mucous m.
membranocartilaginous
membranous
    bronchitis, m.
    cochlea, m.
    croup, m.
    labyrinth, m.
    laryngitis, m.
    pharyngitis, m.
    semicircular canals, m.
    stomatitis, m.
Meniere disease
meningitis
meningoencephalitis mumps
meningo-oculofacial angiomatosis
mental
    audition, m.
    crest, m.
    foramen, m.
    nerve, m.
    point, m.
    prominence, m.
    protuberance, m.
    tubercle, m.
mentalis
    muscle, m.
menthol
mentoanterior
mentobregmatic diameter
mentolabial
menton
mentoparietal
mentoplasty
mentoposterior
mentotransverse
mentum
mephitic
mephitis
mercurial stomatitis
mercurialism
mercury-filled esophageal bougie
Merkel filtrum
Merocel

Merocel *(continued)*
    ear packing, M.
    ear wick, M.
    nasal pack, M.
    nasal tampon, M.
    sponge, M.
merosmia
Merrifield knife
mesenteric sling
mesethmoid
mesial (M)
    angles, m.
    cavity, m.
    drift, m.
    occlusion, m.
    surface, m.
mesially
mesiobuccal (MB)
mesiobuccopulpal (MBP)
mesiobucco-occlusal (MBO)
mesiocervical (MC)
mesioclination
mesioclusion
mesiodens (pl. mesiodentes)
mesiodentes (pl. of mesiodens)
mesiodistal (MD)
mesiogingival (MG)
mesioincisodistal (MID)
mesiolabial (MLA)
mesiolabioincisal (MLAI)
mesiolingual (ML)
mesiolinguoincisal (MLI)
mesiolinguo-occlusal (MLO)
mesiolinguopulpal (MLP)
mesion
mesio-occlusal (MO)
mesio-occlusion
mesio-occludistal (MOD)
mesiopulpal (MP)
mesiopulpolabial (MPLA)
mesiopulpolingual (MPL)
mesioversion
mesobranchial
mesobronchitis
mesocephalic
mesodont

mesodontic
mesodontism
mesoesophagus
mesognathion
mesognathous
mesonasal
mesorrhine
mesostaphyline
mesotaurodontism
mesoturbinal
mesoturbinate
mesotympanum
Messer-Klinger technique
metabolic
    craniopathy, m.
    encephalopathy, m.
metacone
metaconid
metaconule
metafacial angle
metal insert tooth
metallic foreign body
metallizing
metastatic mumps
meter mask
metered dose
methacrylate
methacrylic acid
methyl methacrylate
methylprednisolone
metopantralgia
metopantritis
metopic point
metopion
Metzenbaum
    baby tonsillar scissors, M.
    septum knife, M.
Metzenbaum-Lipsett scissors
Meyer
    disease, M.
    organ, M.
    sinus, M.
Meyer-Schwickerath and Weyers syndrome
MG (mesiogingival)
Michel

Michel *(continued)*
    deformity, M.
    deafness, M.
    rhinoscopic mirror, M.
Michelson bronchoscope
micracusia
MICRINS 2000 microsurgical instruments
microcephaly
microcheilia
microdirect laryngoscopy
microdont
microdontia
microdontism
microgenia
microglossia
micrognathia
    -glossoptosis syndrome, m.
Microinvasive balloon dilator
microlaryngeal
microlaryngoscopic
microlaryngoscopy
micromandible
micromaxilla
microphonic
    cochlear m.
microprosopus
microrhinia
microsmatic
microstomia
microsurgery
microsurgical
microtia
microtubule
microtus
MID (mesioincisodistal)
midbrain deafness
middle
    ear, m.
    ear contents, m.
    ear deafness, m.
    meatus, m.
    turbinate, m.
Middleton adenoid curette
midface
Miege syndrome

migraine
migrainous
migrating
   cheilitis, m.
   tooth, m.
migration
   tooth m.
Mikulicz
   aphthae, M.
   cells, M.
   operation, M.
   pharyngoesophageal reconstruction, M.
   syndrome, M.
   tarsectomy, M.
   tonsillar forceps, M.
Miles
   antral curette, M.
   nasal pouch, M.
milk teeth
Mill-Rose esophageal injector
Millar
   asthma, M.
Millard
   cheiloplasty, M.
   forehead flap, M.
   island flap, M.
   rotation-advancement technique, M.
   -type thimble hook, M.
Millard-Gubler syndrome
milled-in paths
Miller
   colutory, M.
   laryngoscope, M.
   tonsillar dissector, M.
millers' asthma
Millette tonsil knife
milliner's needle
milling-in
mimic tic
miners'
   asthma, m.
   nystagmus, m.
Minamata disease
mineralization
Minerva

Minerva *(continued)*
   plaster collar, M.
   plaster jacket, M.
minimum tension skin lines
miniplate fixation
minor cartilages
Minot-von Willebrand syndrome
Mirault procedure
Mirault-Brown-Blair procedure
mirror
   dental m.
   frontal m.
   head m.
   Glatzel m.
   mouth m.
   nasographic m.
mirror laryngoscope
mirror laryngoscopy
mirror speech
mirror test
Mirschamps sign
mist tent
mistura
Mittlemeyer test
mixed
   aphasia, m.
   deafness, m.
   flora, m.
   hearing loss, m.
MKV (killed-measles vaccine)
ML (mesiolingual)
MLA (mesiolabial)
Mladick ear reconstruction
MLAI (mesiolabioincisal)
MLB (monaural loudness balance)
MLI (mesiolinguoincisal)
MLNS (mucocutaneous lymph node syndrome)
MLO (mesiolinguo-occlusal)
MLP (mesiolinguopulpal)
MMR (measles/mumps/rubella) vaccine
MO (mesio-occlusal)
mobile tooth
mobilization
   stapes, m. of
mobilize

mobilizer
Mobius syndrome
MOD (mesio-occlusodistal)
modified Rethi flying bird incision
modioli (pl. of modiolus)
modiolus (pl. modioli)
Moeller glossitis
Moersch
    bronchoscope, M.
    esophagoscope, M.
    forceps, M.
mogilalia
mogiphonia
Mohr syndrome
Mohs hardness test
moist
    cough, m.
    heat, m.
molar
    impacted m.
    Moon m's
    mulberry m.
    sixth-year m.
    supernumerary m.
    third m.
    twelfth-year m.
molar band
molar teeth
molariform
molaris
    tertius, m.
molding
    border m.
    compression m.
    injection m.
    tissue m.
Mollison mastoid rongeur
Molt
    guillotine, M.
    mouth gag, M.
    mouth prop, M.
Molt-Storz
    guillotine, M.
    tonsillectome, M.
monangle
monaural

monaural *(continued)*
    hearing loss, m.
    loudness balance, m. (MLB)
Mondini
    deafness, M.
    dysplasia, M.
monilial esophagitis
Monks otoplasty
monoblock
    activator, m.
    appliance, m.
monomaxillary
monomorphic adenoma
mononucleosis
monophyodont dentition
monorhinic
Monospot test
monotic
Monson curve
Montefiore tracheal tube
Montgomery
    tracheal cannula system, M.
    T tube, M.
moon
    face, m.
    facies, m.
    -shaped face, m.
    -shaped facies, m.
Moon
    molars, M.
    teeth, M.
Moore-Sullivan technique
Moorehead cheek retractor
Morand foramen
Moraxella
    catarrhalis, M.
morcellize
Morch
    swivel tracheostomy tube
    ventilator, M.
Morel ear
Morel-Fatio blepharoplasty
Morestin otoplasty
Morgagni
    hyperostosis, M.
    sacculus, M.

Morgagni *(continued)*
   sinus, M.
   ventricle, M.
Moritz-Schmidt laryngeal forceps
Morquio disease
Morquio-Ullrich syndrome
Morris biphase fixation apparatus
Morrison-Hurd
   pillar retractor, M.
   tonsillar dissector, M.
morsal
   teeth, m.
Morsch-Retec respirator
morsicatio buccarum
morsulus
mortise
Morton cough
Moss classification
moss-agate sputum
Mosher
   curette, M.
   esophagoscope, M.
   ethmoid punch forceps, M.
   speculum, M.
Moss Mark IV nasal tube
Motais operation
motility
   esophageal m.
motion sickness
motor aphasia
mottled
   appearance, m.
   enamel, m.
   teeth, m.
mottling
moulage
moulding
mount
   x-ray m.
mounting
   split cast m.
Moure esophagoscope
mouse-tooth forceps
Mousseau-Barbin esophageal tube
moustache dressing
mouth

mouth *(continued)*
   Ceylon sore m.
   denture sore m.
   dry m.
   glass-blower's m.
   sore m.
   tapir m.
   trench m.
   white m.
mouth-breather
mouth breathing
mouth cells
mouth gag
mouth prop
mouthrinse
mouthwash
movement
   Bennett m.
   border m.
   border tissue m's
   gliding m.
   hinge m.
   intermediary m's
   intermediate m's
   jaw m.
   Magnan m.
   mandibular m.
   masticatory m's
   opening m.
moving platform fistula test (MPFT)
moxalactam
Mozart ear
MP (mesiopulpal)
MPFT (moving platform fistula test)
MPL (mesiopulpolingual)
MPLA (mesiopulpolabial)
MPS (mucopolysaccharidosis)
Mrazik midfacial osteotomy
MRT Tidal Humidifier
muciform
mucigenous
mucigogue
mucin
muciparous glands
mucitis
Muck

Muck *(continued)*
    tonsillar forceps, M.
    tonsillar hemostat, M.
Muckle-Wells syndrome
mucobuccal fold
mucocele
mucociliary
mucoclasis
mucocutaneous
    flap, m.
    junction, m.
    lymph node syndrome, m. (MLNS)
mucoepidermoid carcinoma
mucogingival
    junction, m.
mucoid
mucolabial
mucolytic
mucomembranous
Mucomyst
mucoperichondrial
mucoperichondrium
mucoperiosteal
    elevator, m.
    flap, m.
    tissue, m.
mucoperiosteum
mucopolysaccharidosis (MPS)
mucopurulence
mucopurulent
    discharge, m.
    drainage, m.
    exudate, m.
    sputum, m.
mucopus
mucopyocele
mucormycosis
mucosa
    alveolar m.
    lingual m.
    masticatory m.
    nasal m.
    oral m.
mucosal
    graft, m.
    surfaces, m.

mucosanguineous
mucosedative
mucoserous
    otitis media, m.
mucosin
mucosis
    otitis, m.
mucositis
mucosocutaneous
mucostatic
mucosus otitis
mucosus
    otitis, m.
mucous
    glands, m.
    membrane, m.
    plug, m.
    retention cyst, m.
    retention phenomenon, m.
    sheets, m.
    threads, m.
mucoviscid
mucoviscidosis
mucro
mucus
    inhibitor, m.
Mueller
    muscle, M.
    tongue blade, M.
Mueller-Laforce adenotome
Mui scientific 6-channel esophageal
    pressure probe
mulberry molar
Mulder angle
Muldoon
    lacrimal dilator, M.
    lid retractor, M.
Mules technique
Muller
    experiment, M.
    muscle, M.
multicuspid
multicuspidate
multidentate
multiple anchorage
multirooted

mumps
   iodine m.
mumps antibody titer
mumps meningitis
mumps meningoencephalitis
mumps virus
Murphy
   endotracheal tube, M.
   tonsillar forceps, M.
musculoaponeurotic
musculoarticular
musculoplasty
Museholdt forceps
music deafness
mussitation
mustache dressing
mustard plaster
Mustarde
   eyelid procedure, M.
   four-flap epicanthal repair, M.
   otoplasty, M.
Mustarde-Furnas otoplasty
mute
mutism
   akinetic m.
   deaf m.
   elective m.
myalgia
myasthenia
   gravis, m.
   laryngis, m.
   neonatal m.
myasthenic
mycelial cluster
mycomyringitis
mycoplasma
mycosis
   leptothrica, m.
mycotic
   stomatitis, m.
Myerson
   antrum trocar, M.
   miniature laryngeal biopsy forceps, M.
   saw, M.
myiasis
Myles

Myles *(continued)*
   adenotome, M.
   antral curette, M.
   forceps, M.
   guillotine adenotome, M.
   nasal punch, M.
   sinus antral cannula, M.
   snare, M.
   speculum, M.
   tonsillectome, M.
mylohyoid
   line, m.
   muscle, m.
   ridge, m.
   vessel, m.
mylohyoideus
mylopharyngeal
mylopharyngeus
myoblastoma
myochorditis
myoclonus
myocutaneous
   flap, m.
myofasciitis
myognathus
myoneural junction
myopathic
   facies, m.
myopathy
myositis
myringa
myringectomy
myringitis
   bullosa, m.
   bullous m.
myringodectomy
myringodermatitis
myringomycosis
   aspergillina, m.
myringoplasty
   knife, m.
myringorupture
myringoscope
myringoscopy
myringostapediopexy
myringotome

myringotome *(continued)*
   knife, m.
myringotomy
   incision, m.
   knife, m.
myrinx
myrtiform fossa
myxadenitis
   labialis, m.
myxadenoma
myxangitis
myxasthenia

myxedema
myxedematoid
myxedematous
myxiosis
myxoid
myxoma (pl. myxomata)
myxomata (pl. of myxoma)
myxomatous
myxopoiesis
myxorrhea
myxovirus

Additional entries

N

N2O (nitrous oxide)
Nadbath akinesia
Naegeli syndrome
Nager acrofacial dysostosis
Nance leeway space
nanoid enamel
nape of neck
    flap, n.
napkin-ring stenosis
nares (pl. of naris)
naris (pl. nares)
    anterior n.
    external n.
    internal n.
    posterior n.
nasal
    airway, n.
    airway obstruction, n.
    ala, n.
    allergy, n.
    antral window, n.
    antrum, n.
    aperture, n.
    arch, n.
    asthma, n.
    balloon, n.
    bistoury, n.
    bleeding, n.
    bone, n.
    border, n.
    breathing, n.
    bridge, n.
    calculus, n.
    canal, n.
    canthus, n.
    cartilage, n.
    cartilage-cutting board, n.
    cartilage-holding forceps, n.
    catarrh, n.
    catheter, n.
    cautery, n.
    cavity, n.
    chamber, n.

nasal *(continued)*
    chisel, n.
    cleft, n.
    concha, n.
    congestion, n,
    contour, n.
    crest, n.
    culture, n.
    curette, n.
    -cutting forceps, n.
    decongestant, n.
    deformity, n.
    discharge, n.
    dome, n.
    douche, n.
    drainage, n.
    dressing forceps, n.
    drip pad, n.
    duct, n.
    elevator, n.
    eminence, n.
    endoscopy telescope, n.
    feeding, n.
    filtration, n.
    flaring, n.
    forceps, n.
    fossa, n.
    gavage, n.
    gouge, n.
    grasping forceps, n.
    height, n.
    hook, n.
    hump, n.
    hump-cutting forceps, n.
    index, n.
    insertion, n.
    insufflation, n.
    intubation, n.
    knife, n.
    laminae, n.
    line, n.
    meatus, n.
    mucosa, n.

nasal *(continued)*
    mucous blanket, n.
    notch of maxilla, n.
    obstruction, n.
    oxygen, n.
    packing, n.
    passage, n.
    pit, n.
    polyp, n.
    polyp hook, n.
    polypectomy, n.
    probe, n.
    prongs, n.
    punch, n.
    pyramid, n.
    rasp, n.
    reconstruction, n.
    reflex, n.
    resistance, n.
    retractor, n.
    rongeur, n.
    saw, n.
    scissors, n.
    septal cartilage, n.
    septoplasty, n.
    septum, n.
    septum reconstruction, n. (NSR)
    sill, n.
    sinus, n.
    smear, n.
    snare, n.
    speculum, n.
    spine, n.
    splint, n.
    spray, n.
    spur, n.
    stent, n.
    steroids, n.
    strut, n.
    suction, n.
    suction tip, n.
    suture, n.
    swivel knife, n.
    tampon, n.
    tamponade, n.
    tip rotation, n.

nasal *(continued)*
    trephine, n.
    truss, n.
    tube, n.
    turbinate, n.
    vault, n.
    vestibule, n.
    vestibulitis, n.
    washings, n.
    width, n.
Nasalide
nasalis
nasality
nasioiniac
nasion
    postcondylare plane, n.
nasitis
Nasmyth membrane
nasoalveolar cyst
nasoantral
    window, n.
nasoantritis
nasoantrostomy
nasobronchial
nasociliaris
nasociliary
nasoendotracheal
nasoesophageal
nasofrontal
nasofrontalis
nasogastric (NG)
    catheter, n.
    feeding tube, n.
    intubation, n.
    suction, n.
    tube, n.
nasograph
nasographic mirror
nasojejunal (NJ)
    feeding, n.
    feeding solution, n.
nasolabial
    crease, n.
    droop, n.
    flap, n.
    fold, n.

nasolabial *(continued)*
    junction, n.
    lymph node, n.
nasolabialis
nasolacrimal
    canal, n.
    duct, n.
    tube, n.
nasology
nasomandibular
    fixation, n.
nasomanometer
nasomaxillary
nasomental
    reflex, n.
nasonnement
naso-optic
naso-oral
nasopalatine
    canal, n.
    nerve, n.
    pad cyst, n.
    plexus of Woodruoff, n.
    recess, n.
nasopharyngeal (NP)
    applicator, n.
    bursitis, n.
    carcinoma, n. (NPC)
    duct, n.
    electrode, n.
    regurgitation, n.
    pack, n.
    retractor, n.
    secretions, n.
    speculum, n.
    torticollis, n.
    tube, n.
nasopharyngitis
nasopharyngography
nasopharyngolaryngoscope
nasopharyngoscope
nasopharynx
nasopineal angle
nasorostral
nasoscope
nasoseptal

nasoseptal *(continued)*
    deviation, n.
    reconstruction, n.
nasoseptitis
nasosinusitis
nasospinale
nasostat
nasotracheal (NT)
    catheter, n.
    intubation, n.
    suction, n.
    tube, n.
nasoturbinal
    concha, n.
nasus
    externus, n.
natal teeth
natural teeth
nausea
nauseant
nauseated
nauseous
navel
    enamel n.
Nebinger-Praun operation
nebulization
nebulized mist
nebulizer
neck
    bull n.
    condyloid process of mandible, n. of
    dental n.
    Madelung n.
    malleus, n. of
    mandible, n. of
    stiff n.
    tooth, n. of
    turkey gobbler n.
    webbed n.
    wry n.
neck conformer
neck dissection
neck crease
neck flap
neck lift
neck stiffness

necklace
    Casal n.
necrosis
necrotic
necrotizing
    external otitis, n. (NEO)
    ulcerative gingitivis, n, (NUG)
needlepoint
    electrocautery, n.
    tracing, n.
Negus
    bronchoscope, N.
    mouth gag, N
Negus-Broyles bronchoscope
Neivert
    dissector, N.
    knife, N.
    nasal osteotome, N.
    nasal polyp hook, N.
    retractor, N.
    tonsil snare, N.
Nelaton otoplasty
NEMD (nonspecific esophageal motility disorder)
NEO (necrotizing external otitis)
neoglottic
neoglottis
neonatal
    lines, n.
    teeth, n.
Neo-Synephrine
neoturbinate
nerve conduction
    deafness, n.
nerve deafness
nervous asthma
Neubauer artery
Neumann
    method, N.
    sheath, N.
neural
    deafness, n.
    pathway, n.
neuralgia
    facial n.
    Fothergill n.

neuralgia *(continued)*
    glossopharyngeal n.
    Harris migrainous n.
    mandibular joint n.
    migrainous n.
    nasociliary n.
    occipital n.
    otic n.
    retrobulbar n.
    Sluder n.
    sphenopalatine n.
    supraorbital n.
    trifacial n.
    trigeminal n.
    vidian n.
neuralgic
neuralgiform
neurapraxia
neurasthenic asthma
neurilemmoma
neuritic
neuritis
neurofibroma
neurofibromatous
neurogenic
neurolabyrinthitis
neuroma
    acoustic n.
neuronitis
neurophonia
neurotologist
neurotology
neutrocclusion
Neville
    tracheal prosthesis, N.
    tracheobronchial prosthesis, N.
nevoid
nevus
    Naegeli, n. of
Nevyas drape retractor
New tracheal hook
New-Lambotte osteotome
New Orleans Eye and Ear forceps
New York Eye and Ear
    cannula, N.
    forceps, N.

Newhart
   incus hook, N.
   mallet, N.
Newkirk mouth gag
Ney procedure
Ney-Chayes attachment
NG (nasogastric)
nib
niche
   enamel n.
Nicolet Nerve Integrity Monitor-2 (NIM-2)
nicotine-stained teeth
nicotinic acid
nictitating spasm
nidus of infection
night
   guard, n.
   sweats, n.
NightBird nasal CPAP
nigrities
   linguae, n.
NIM-2 (Nicolet Nerve Integrity Monitor-2)
Niro arch bar
Nissen fundoplication
niter
   paper, n.
nitre
nitrous oxide (N2O)
NJ (nasojejunal)
   feeding, N.
   tube, N.
nocturnal vertigo
nodal
nodding spasm
node
   buccal lymph n.
   buccinator lymph n.
   Delphian n.
   facial lymph n's
   lymph n.
   malar lymph n.
   mandibular lymph n.
   mastoid lymph n's
   nasolabial lymph n.

node *(continued)*
   paratracheal lymph n's
   parotid lymph n's
   prelaryngeal n.
   pretracheal lymph n's
   retroauricular lymph n's
   retropharyngeal lymph n's
   Rosenmuller n.
   singer's n.
   submandibular lymph n's
   submental lymph n's
   teacher's n.
   thyroid lymph n's
   tracheal lymph n's
   tracheobronchial lymph n's
nodose ganglion
nodular
nodule
   Bohn n's
   singers' n.
   teachers' n.
   vestigial n.
   vocal n.
   warm n.
noise
   white n.
noise pollution
noma
nominal aphasia
nonacoustic labyrinth
nonairflow rhinitis
nonallergic
   rhinitis, n.
nonfluent aphasia
nonocclusion
nonproductive cough
nonrebreathing mask
nonspecific esophageal motility disorder (NEMD)
nonus (eleventh cranial nerve)
nonvital tooth
Noonan syndrome
normal flora
nose
   beaked n.
   cleft n.

nose *(continued)*
   dished n.
   external n.
   flattened n.
   hammer n.
   polly-beak n.
   potato n.
   pug n.
   Roman n.
   saddle n.
   saddle-back n.
   swayback n.
nose-blowing
nose-breather
nose-breathing
nose-bridge prosthesis
nose drops
nose job (rhinoplasty)
nose-picking
nose plug
nose ring
nosebleed
nosebrain
nostril
   elevator, n.
   reflex, n.
notch
   ethmoidal n.
   frontal n.
   jugular n.
   labial n.
   lacrimal n.
   mandibular n.
   mastoid n.
   maxilla, n. of
   nasal n.
   nasolacrimal n.
   palatine bone, n. of
   parotid n.
   rivinian n.
   Rivinus, n. of
   sigmoid n.
   sphenopalatine n.
   thyroid n.
   tympanic n.
Nottingham introducer

Novafil suture
Noyes nasal dressing forceps
Noyes-Shambaugh scissors
NP (nasopharyngeal)
   culture, N.
NPC (nasopharyngeal carcinoma)
NPO (nothing by mouth)
NSR (nasal septal reconstruction)
NT (nasotracheal)
nu angle
nucha
nuchal
   adenopathy, n.
   cord, n.
   ligament, n.
   line, n.
   planum, n.
   rigidity, n.
nucleus
   ambiguous n.
   auditory n.
   Bechterew n.
   Bekhterev n.
   cochlear n.
   Deiters n.
   facial motor n.
   habenular n.
   hypoglossal n.
   masticatory n.
   motor n. of trigeminal nerve
   oculomotor n.
   Perlia, n. of
   principal trigeminal sensory n.
   salivary n.
   sensory n. of trigeminal nerve
   trigeminal spinal n.
   vestibular n.
Nucofed
Nuel space
NUG (necrotizing ulcerative gingivitis)
Nuhn glands
numb lip syndrome
nummular sputum
nutcracker esophagus
Nuva-Seal
nystagmoid

nystagmus
    amaurotic n.
    ambylopic n.
    ataxic n.
    aural n.
    caloric n.
    central n.
    Cheyne n.
    Cheyne-Stokes n.
    congenital n.
    congenital hereditary n.
    convergence n.
    convergence-retraction n.
    disjunctive n.
    dissociated n.
    downbeat n.
    electrical n.
    end-position n.
    fixation n.
    galvanic n.
    gaze n.
    jerk n.
    labyrinthine n.
    latent n.
    lateral n.
    miner's n.
    ocular n.

nystagmus *(continued)*
    opticokinetic n.
    optokinetic n.
    oscillating n.
    palatal n.
    paretic n.
    pendular n.
    periodic alternating n.
    positional n.
    railroad n.
    resilient n.
    retraction n.
    rhythmic n.
    rotatory n.
    secondary n.
    see-saw n.
    spontaneous n.
    undulatory n.
    unilateral n.
    vertical n.
    vestibular n.
    vibratory n.
    visual n.
    voluntary n.
nystagmus-myoclonus
nystaxis

Additional entries

O

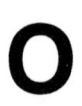

Oakey technique
OAV (oculoauriculovertebral)
obligate
    mouth-breather, o.
    nose-breather, o.
oblique ramus sliding technique
obmutescence
obstructed airway
obstruction
    airway o.
    nasal airway o.
obstructive
    airways disease, o.
    sleep apnea (OSA), o.
obturation
    canal o.
obturator
    appliance, o.
Obwegeser
    sagittal mandibular osteotomy procedure, O.
    splitting chisel, O.
Obwegeser-Dal Pont sagittal osteotomy
OC (occlusocervical)
occipital
    anchorage, o.
occipitofacial
occipitofrontal diameter
occipitomastoid
occipitomental diameter
occiput
occlude
occluder
occluding centric relation record
occlusal
    cavity, o.
    contact, o.
    contouring, o.
    force, o.
    glide, o.
    guide, o.
    harmony, o.
    load, o.

occlusal *(continued)*
    mold, o.
    pattern, o.
    plane, o.
    rest bar, o.
    surface, o.
    wear, o.
occlusion
    abnormal o.
    acentric o.
    adjusted o.
    afunctional o.
    anatomic o.
    anterior o.
    balanced o.
    buccal o.
    central o.
    centric o.
    coronary o.
    dental o.
    distal o.
    eccentric o.
    edge-to-edge o.
    end-to-end o.
    functional o.
    habitual o.
    hyperfunctional o.
    ideal o.
    labial o.
    lateral o.
    lingual o.
    mechanically-balanced o.
    mesial o.
    neutral o.
    normal o.
    pathogenic o.
    posterior o.
    postnormal o.
    prenormal o.
    protrusive o.
    retrusive o.
    spherical form of o.
    terminal o.

occlusion *(continued)*
   traumatic o.
   traumatogenic o.
   working o.
occlusion laryngostenosis
occlusive
occlusocervical (OC)
occlusometer
occlusometry
occlusorehabilitation
occupational exposure
   deafness, o.
   hearing loss, o.
   myopathy, o.
Ocean nasal spray
Ochsenbein gingivectomy
ocular nystagmus
oculoauricular dysplasia
oculoauriculovertebral (OAV) dysplasia
oculodentodigital (ODD) dysplasia
oculodento-osseous (ODO) dysplasia
oculofacial
oculomandibulofacial
oculomotor
oculonasal
oculopharyngeal
   reflex, o.
oculozygomatic
   line, o.
odaxesmus
ODD (oculodentodigital)
ODO (oculodento-osseous)
odontagra
odontalgia
   phantom o.
odontalgic
odontatrophy
odontectomy
odonterism
odontexis
odontia
odontiatrogenic
odontic
odontitis
odontoameloblastoma
odontoblast

odontoblastoma
odontobothrion
odontobothritis
odontocele
odontochirurgical
odontoclamis
odontoclasis
odontoclast
odontodynia
odontogen
odontogenic
   fibroma, o.
   fibromyxoma, o.
   fibrosarcoma, o.
   keratocyst, o.
   tumor, o.
odontogenesis
   imperfecta, o.
odontogenetic
odontogenic
odontogenous
odontogeny
odontogram
odontograph
odontography
odontoiatria
odontoid
   apophysis, o.
   fracture, o.
   ligaments, o.
   process, o.
   projection, o.
   vertebra, o.
   view, o.
odontolith
odontolithiasis
odontologist
odontology
odontolysis
odontoma
   adamantinum, o.
   ameloblastic o.
   composite o.
   coronal o.
   coronary o.
   dilated o.

odontoma *(continued)*
   embryoplastic o.
   fibrous o.
   follicular o.
   mixed o.
   radicular o.
odontonecrosis
odontonomy
odontopathic
odontopathy
odontoperiosteum
odontophobia
odontoplasty
odontoprisis
odontoradiography
odontorrhagia
odontoschism
odontoscopy
odontoseisis
odontosis
odontotheca
odontotherapy
odontotomy
odontotripsis
odynacusis
odynophagia
oesophageal
OFD (oral-facial-digital or orofaciodigital)
ogo
Ogston-Luc operation
Ogura forceps
Ohio Bubble Humidifier
oil of cloves
OKN (optokinetic nystagmus)
OKN's symmetric
olfact
olfactie
olfaction
olfactism
olfactive angle
olfactology
olfactometer
olfactometry
olfactory
   anesthesia, o.

olfactory *(continued)*
   angle, o.
   areas, o.
   brain, o.
   bulb, o.
   canal, o.
   cells, o.
   cleft, o.
   cortex, o.
   esthesioneuroma, o.
   fasciculus, o.
   foramen, o.
   gland, o.
   groove, o.
   gyrus, o.
   hair, o.
   islands, o.
   labyrinth, o.
   lobe, o.
   membrane, o.
   nasal sulcus, o.
   nerve, o.
   neuroblastoma, o.
   organ, o.
   pit, o.
   stria, o.
   sulcus, o.
   tract, o.
   trigone, o.
   tubercle, o.
olfactus
oligodontia
olive-tip catheter
Olivecrona
   endaural rongeur, O.
   guillotine scissors, O.
   mastoid rongeur, O.
Oliver sign
olivocochlear bundle of Rasmussen
Ollier-Thiersch graft
olophonia
Olympus
   bronchoscope, O.
   ENF-P2 flexible laryngoscope, O.
   esophagofiberscope, O.
   flexible ENT scope, O.

OM (otitis media)
Ombredanne otoplasty
OME (otitis media with effusion)
omental free-flap transfer
omeprazole
O meridian
OMM (ophthalmomandibulomelic)
Ommaya CSF reservoir
Omnipaque
omohyoid muscle
oncocytoma
onlay
    graft, o.
opalescent dentin
opaque
OPD (otopalatodigital) syndrome
open
    bite, o.
    -face crown, o.
    -flap technique, o.
    -mouth odontoid view, o.
    -mouth scan, o.
    reduction and internal fixation, o. (ORIF)
    -sky technique, o.
opening axis
operating
    microscope, o.
    otoscope, o.
opercula (pl. of operculum)
opercular
operculectomy
operculitis
operculum (pl. opercula)
ophryospinal angles
ophthalmomandibulomelic (OMM) dysplasia
ophthalmoplegia
opisthiobasial
opisthion
opisthionasial
opisthocranion
opisthogenia
opisthognathism
opisthotic
opportunistic

opportunistic *(continued)*
    infection, o.
    organism, o.
optic
    aphasia, o.
    nerve, o.
optical
    axis, o.
    esophagoscope, o.
    laryngoscope, o.
opticonasion
optokinetic nystagmus (OKN)
optophone
ora (pl. of os)
orad
oral
    agent, o.
    antibiotic, o.
    arch, o.
    candidiasis, o.
    cavity, o.
    contents, o.
    decongestant, o.
    endotracheal tube, o.
    fistula, o.
    flora, o.
    forceps, o.
    habit, o.
    hygiene, o.
    intubation, o.
    mucosa, o.
    panendoscope, o.
    passages, o.
    pharynx, o.
    restorative surgery, o.
    route, o.
    screw mouth gag, o.
    screw tongue depressor, o.
    secretions, o.
    speculum mouth gag, o.
    thrush, o.
    tori, o.
    tuberculosis, o.
    vestibule, o.
orale
orality

oralogy
oral-facial-digital (OFD)
orbicular
   bone, o.
   process, o.
orbiculare
orbiculus
   oculi, o.
   oris, o.
orbit (pl. orbitae)
orbitae (pl. of orbit)
orbital
   abscess, o.
   cellulitis, o.
   crest, o.
   floor, o.
   floor fracture, o.
   plate, o.
   ridge, o.
   rim, o.
   roof, o.
   step-off, o.
orbitale
orbitalis
orbitography
orbitomeatal
orbitonasal
orbitosphenoid
orbitotemporal
orbitotomy
organ
   acoustic o.
   cement o.
   Corti, o. of
   enamel o.
   gustatory o.
   Jacobson, o. of
   mastication, o's of
   olfactory o.
   Ruffini, o. of
   special sense o's
   spiral o.
   vestibulocochlear o's
   vomeronasal o.
   Y o.
organic deafness

organum
   auditus, o.
   gustus, o.
   olfactus, o.
   spirale, o.
   vestibulocochleare, o.
   vomeronasale, o.
ORIF (open reduction and internal fixation)
orifacial angle
orifice
orificial
oroantral
   fistula, o.
orofacial
   fistula, o.
orofaciodigital (OFD)
orogastric
orolingual
oromandibular
   dystonia, o.
oromaxillary
oronasal
   fistula, o.
oropharyngeal
   achalasia, o.
   airway, o.
   isthmus, o.
   pack, o.
   partition, o.
   tularemia, o.
oropharyngeus
oropharynx
   proper, o.
orotracheal
   tube, o.
orthodentin
orthodontia
orthodontics
   corrective o.
   interceptive o.
   preventive o.
   prophylactic o.
   surgical o.
orthodontist
orthodontology

orthognathia
orthognathic
orthognathics
orthognathous
orthopantogram
orthopantograph
Orthopantomograph
orthopedics
    dentofacial o.
    function jaw o.
orthotic
orthotics
orthotist
Orticochea technique
os (pl. ora)
    epitympanicum, o.
    ethmoidale, o.
    frontale, o.
    hyoideum, o.
    interparietale, o.
    lacrimale, o.
    mastoideum, o.
    nasale, o.
    occipitale, o.
    odontoideum, o.
    orbiculare, o.
    palatinum, o.
    parietale, o.
    sphenoidale, o.
    temporale, o.
    unguis, o.
    zygomaticum, o.
OSA (obstructive sleep apnea)
oscillating
    nystagmus, o.
    saw, o.
Osler-Weber-Rendu symdrome
OSMED (otospondylomegaepiphyseal dysplasia)
osmometer
osmonosology
osmoscope
osphresiology
osphresiometer
osphresis
osphretic

osseointegrated implant
osseous
    labyrinth, o.
osseosonometry
ossicle
    auditory o.'s
    Bertin, o.'s of
    Riolin o.'s
    sphenoturbinal o.'s
ossicula (pl. of ossiculum)
    auditus, o.
ossicular
    chain, o.
    disarticulation, o.
    replacement prosthesis, o.
    repositioning, o.
    system, o.
ossiculectomy
ossiculotomy
ossiculum (pl. ossicula)
ossification
ossified
ossify
ossiphone
Ossoff-Karlen laryngoscope
osteoacusis
osteodentin
osteodentinoma
osteodysplasty
    Melnick and Needles, o. of
osteofluorosis
osteogenic
osteogenesis
    imperfecta, o.
osteoma
osteomeatal sinus tract
osteon
osteonosus
osteo-odontoma
osteoperiostitis
osteopetrosis
osteophony
osteoplastic
    flap, o.
    frontal sinus procedure, o.
    rhinoplasty, o.

osteosclerosis
osterosclerotic
osteoseptum
osteosynthesis
osteotome
osteotomy
    cut, o.
osteotympanic conduction
ostiomeatal sinus disease
ostium
    eustachian tube o.
    maxillare o.
    pharyngeal o.
    pharyngeum tubae auditivae, o.
    tympanicum tubae auditivae, o.
Ostrum
    antrum punch-tip forceps, O.
    nose punch, O.
Ostrum-Furst syndrome
otacoustic
otagra
otalgia
    dentalis, o.
    geniculate o.
    intermittens, o.
    reflex o.
    tabetic o.
otalgic
otantritis
OTC (over-the-counter)
otectomy
othelcosis
othematoma
othemorrhea
othygroma
otiatrics
otic
    capsule, o.
    cerebral abscess, o.
    ganglion, o.
    grandion, o.
    periotic shunt, o.
    vesicle, o.
oticodinia
otitic
    barotrauma, o.

otitic *(continued)*
    hydrocephalus, o.
otitis
    adhesive o. media
    aero-o.
    aviation o.
    chronic adhesive o.
    crouposa, o.
    desquamativa, o.
    diphtheritica, o.
    externa circumscripta, o.
    externa diffusa, o.
    externa furunculosa, o.
    externa hemorrhagica, o.
    externa mycotica, m.
    fibro-osseous o.
    furuncular o.
    haemorrhagica, o.
    interna, o.
    labyrinthica, o.
    mastoidea, o.
    media catarrhalis, o.
    media with effusion, o. (OME)
    media purulenta o.
    media sclerotica, o.
    media serosa, o.
    media suppurativa, o.
    mesia vasomotorica, o.
    mucosis o.
    mucosus o.
    mycotica, o.
    necrotizing external o.
    parasitica, o.
    purulent o.
    sclerotica, o.
    secretory o. media
otoacoustic
otoantritis
otoblennorrhea
otocatarrh
otocephalus
otocephaly
otocerebritis
otocleisis
otoconia (pl. of otoconium)
otoconite

otoconium (pl. of otoconia)
otocranial
otocranium
otocyst
otodynia
otoencephalitis
otoganglion
otogenic
otogenous
otography
otohemineurasthenia
otolaryngologist
otolaryngology
otolite
otolith
otolithiasis
otolithic membrane
otologic
otologist
otology
otomandibular dysostosis
otomassage
otomastoiditis
otomicroscope
Oto-Microscope
otomicroscopy
otomucormycosis
otomyasthenia
Otomyces
 hageni, O.
 purpureus, O.
otomycosis
 aspergillina, o.
otomyiasis
otoncus
otonecrectomy
otonecronectomy
otoneuralgia
otoneurasthenia
otoneurologic
otoneurology
otopalatodigital (OPD) syndrome
otopathic
otopathy
otopexy
otopharyngeal

otopharyngeal *(continued)*
 tube, o.
otophone
otopiesis
otoplasty
otopolypus
otopyorrhea
otopyosis
otor
otorhinolaryngologist
otorhinolaryngology
otorhinologist
otorhinology
otorrhagia
otorrhea
 cerebrospinal fluid o.
otosalpinx
otosclerectomy
otoscleronectomy
otosclerosis
 cochlear o.
 fenestral o.
otosclerotic
 processes, o.
otoscope
otoscopic
otoscopy
otosis
otospondylomegaepiphyseal dysplasia
 (OSMED)
otospongiosis
otosteal
otosteon
ototome drill
ototomy
ototoxic
 deafness, o.
ototoxicity
Ottolengui bimaxillary procedure
OU (each eye)
oulectomy
oulitis
outer ear
outfracture
outpouching
oval esophagoscope

oval window (OW)
    hook, o.
    niche, o.
    reflex, o.
over-and-out cheek flap
over-the-counter (OTC)
    medication, o.
overbite
    reduction, o.
overclosure
overdenture
overeruption
overextension
overhang
Overholt-Jackson bronchoscope
overjet
    reduction, o.
overjut
overlap
overlay
    crown, o.
    denture, o.
override
overriding

OW (oval window)
Owens
    lines, O.
    position, O.
    procedure, O.
    view, O.
Oxford cleft palate repair
oximeter
oximetry
oxyecoia
oxygen
    cisternography, o.
    mask, o.
oxygenation
oxygeusia
oxyosmia
oxyosphresia
oxyphilic adenoma
oxyphonia
ozena
    laryngis, o.
ozenous
ozostomia

Additional entries

P

P (pulpal)
PA (pulpoaxial)
pachycheilia
pachyglossia
pachygnathous
pachynsis
pachyotia
pachyrhinic
pacifier
pack
    anterior throat p.
    nasal p.
    periodontal p.
    posterior throat p.
    throat p.
pack-year smoking history
pad
    buccal fat p.
    fat p.
    gum p's
    occlusal p.
    Passavant p.
    retromolar p.
    sucking p.
paddle
    skin, p. of
    spring, p.
Padgett dermatome
Padgett-Hood electrodermatome
Page
    tonsillar forceps, P.
    tonsillar knife, P.
Pagenstecher technique
pagetoid
    deafness, p.
    hearing loss, p.
palata (pl. of palatum)
palatal
    abscess, p.
    arch, p.
    bar, p.
    cleft, p.
    index, p.

palatal *(continued)*
    linguoplate, p.
    myoclonus, p.
    nystagmus, p.
    process of maxilla, p.
    pushback procedure, p.
    reflex, p.
    shelf, p.
    vault, p.
palate
    artificial p.
    bony p.
    bony hard p.
    cleft p.
    falling p.
    gothic p.
    hard p.
    pendulous p.
    premaxillary p.
    primary p.
    secondary p.
    smoker's p.
    soft p.
palate bones
palate elevator
palate hook
palate lengthening
palate pusher hook
palate retractor
palatiform
palatine
    aponeurosis, p.
    arch, p.
    artery, p.
    bone, p.
    canal, p.
    cells, p.
    crest, p.
    durum, p.
    folds, p.
    foramen, p.
    muscles, p.
    nerves, p.

palatine *(continued)*
  notch, p.
  process, p.
  protuberance, p.
  raphe, p.
  reflex, p.
  spine, p.
  suture, p.
  tonsil, p.
  uvula, p.
  velum, p.
palatitis
palatoethmoidal
palatoglossal
  arch, p.
palatoglossus
palatognathous
palatograph
palatography
palatomaxillary
  arch, p.
  canal, p.
palatomyograph
palatomyography
palatonasal
palatopagus
palatopharyngeal
  arch, p.
  muscle, p.
  sphincter, p.
palatopharyngeus
  muscle, p.
palatopharyngoplasty
palatoplasty
palatoplegia
palatoproximal
palatorrhaphy
palatosalpingeus
palatoschisis
palatostaphylinus
palatouvularis
palatovaginal canal
palatum (pl. palata)
  durum, p.
  fissum, p.
  molle, p.

palatum (pl. palata) *(continued)*
  ogivale, p.
  osseum, p.
palisade
palisading
pallanesthesia
pallesthesia
pallhypesthesia
pallor
palm-chin reflex
palmomental reflex
palpebra (pl. palpebrae)
palpebrae (pl. of palpebra)
palpebral
  arch, p.
  bags, p.
  commissure, p.
  fissure, p.
  fold, p.
palpebralis
palpebrate
palpebritis
palpebronasal
palsy
  Bell p.
  cerebral p.
  facial p.
  progressive supranuclear p.
PAM (potential acuity meter)
PAN (periodic alternating nystagmus)
Panas ptosis procedure
Pang forceps
Panje voice button
Pankey-Mann-Schuyler procedure
panoral
  radiography, p.
panoramic radiography
Panorex
  films, P.
  view, P.
panotitis
panseptum
pansinuitis
pansinusectomy
pansinusitis
pantomography

Pantopaque
panturbinate
Panus technique
Paparella
   curette, P.
   elevator, P.
   fenestrometer, P.
   otologic surgery elevator
   pick, P.
   tube, P.
Paparella-McCabe crurotomy saw
papilla (pl. papillae)
   acoustic p.
   conical p.
   corium, p. of
   dental p.
   filiform p.
   filiformes, p.
   foliate p.
   foliatae, p.
   fungiform p.
   fungiformes, p.
   gingival p.
   gustatory p.
   incisive p.
   interdental p.
   interproximal p.
   lacrimal p.
   lenticular p.
   lingual p.
   linguales, p.
   palatine p.
   parotid p.
   parotidea, p.
   sublingual p.
   taste p.
   tongue, p. of
papillae (pl. of papilla)
papillary
   gingiva, p.
   gingivitis, p.
papilledema
papilloma
   inverted p.
   squamous p.
Papillon-Lefevre syndrome

papula
papular
paracentesis
paracoccidioidomycosis
paracone
paraconid
paracousis
paracusia
   acris, p.
   duplicata, p.
   loci, p.
   willisiana, p.
paracusis
   Willis, p. of
paradental
paradentitis
paradentium
paradentosis
paradoxic
   deafness, p.
   hearing loss, p.
paraequilibrium
paraesophageal
   hernia, p.
   line, p.
parageusia
paraglossa
paraglossia
paraglossitis
paragnathus
parahiatal
   hernia, p.
parainfluenza
parakeratosis
paralalia
paralysis
   Bell's p.
   brachiofacial p.
   crossed p.
   diphtheritic p.
   facial p.
   glossolabial p.
   Gubler p.
   histrionic p.
   labial p.
   mimetic p.

168 paralysis

paralysis *(continued)*
    phonetic p.
    postdiphtheritic p.
    posticus, p.
    supranuclear p.
    vocal cord p.
paralytic
    rabies, p.
paralyzing vertigo
paramastoid
    process, p.
paramastoiditis
parameatal
paramolar
paramyotonia
    congenita, p.
paranasal
    sinuses, p.
paraoral
parapertussis
parapharyngeal
    abscess, p.
paraphonia
    puberum, p.
pararhizoclasia
pararthria
parasaccular
parasinoidal
    lacunae, p.
paraspasmus
    faciale, p.
parasymphyseal
parasymphysis
parathyroid
    adenoma, p.
    extract, p.
    insufficiency, p.
parathyroidal
parathyroidectomize
parathyroidectomy
parathyroprival
parathyroprivous
parathyrotoxicosis
parathyrotropic
paratonsillar
paratracheal

paratracheal *(continued)*
    line, p.
    lymph nodes, p.
    stripe, p.
parched
    lips, p.
    mouth, p.
Par-Decon
parenchyma
parenchymal
paretic nystagmus
paries (pl. parietes)
    externus ductus cochlearis, p.
    jugularis cavi tympani, p.
    labyrinthicus cavi tympani, p.
    mastoideus cavi tympani, p.
    medialis orbitae, p.
    membranaceus cavi tympani, p.
    membranaceus tracheae, p.
    tegmentalis cavi tympani, p.
    tympanicus ductus cochlearis, p.
    vestibularis ductus cochlearis, p.
parietal
parietes (pl. of paries)
parietitis
parietofrontal
parietomastoid
parieto-occipital
    aphasia, p.
parieto-orbital
parietosphenoid
parietosquamosal
parietotemporal
Parkes
    hump gouge, P.
    nasal raspatory, P.
Parkhill otoplasty
paroccipital
parodontal
parodontid
paradontitis
parodontium
parolfactory
    area, p.
paroral
    membrane, p.

parorexia
parosmia
parosphresia
parosphresis
parotic
parotid
    calculus, p.
    duct, p.
    gland, p.
    lymph nodes, p.
    nerve, p.
    notch, p.
    plexus, p.
    saliva, p.
    stone, p.
parotidean
parotidectomy
parotideomasseterica
    fascia, p.
parotiditis
parotidoscirrhus
parotidosclerosis
parotin
parotitis
    epidemic p.
    phlegmonosa, p.
    postoperative p.
    staphylococcal p.
parotofacial
paroxysm
paroxysmal
    cough, p.
    nocturnal dyspnea, p. (PND)
    sneezing, p.
parrot
    -beak shape of distal esophagus, p.
    jaw, p.
    tongue, p.
Parry's disease
pars
    buccalis hypophyseos, p.
    flaccida portion of tympanic membrane, p. (PFLAC)
    mastoideaossis temporalis, p.
    petrosis ossis temporalis, p.
    tensa membranae tympani, p.

pars *(continued)*
    tympanica ossis temporalis, p.
partial
    denture, p.
    ossicular reconstructive prosthesis, p. (PORP)
    ossicular replacement prosthesis, p. (PORP)
    rebreathing mask, p.
    veneer crown, p.
partition
    oropharyngeal p.
Partsch
    marsupialization, P.
    operation, P.
parulis
Par-Decon
Passavant
    bar, P.
    cushion, P.
    fold, P.
    pad, P.
    ridge, P.
passive lingual arch
pass-over humidifier
paste carrier
pastille
patency
patent
Paterson
    cannula, P.
    forceps, P.
    syndrome, P.
Paterson-Brown Kelly syndrome
Paterson-Kelly syndrome
path
    condyle p.
    incisor p.
    insertion, p. of
    lateral condyle p.
    milled-in p's
    occlusal p.
pathemic aphasia
pathfinder
    broach, p.
pathodontia

Patil stereotactic system
Pattee auditory canal prosthesis
pattern wax
Patterson procedure
Patton nasal speculum
Paulus Titanium chin plate system
pavilion of ear
PB (pulpobuccal)
PBA (pulpobuccoaxial)
PD (pulpodistal)
PD&P (postural drainage and percussion)
PE (pharyngoesophageal)
peacock sound
peak-and-trough levels
peak-flow meter
pearl
   Bohn p's
   enamel p's
   Epstein p's
   gouty p.
pebbled texture
   Laennec p's
Peck-Vienna nasal speculum
pectoralis major myocutaneous flap
pectoriloquous bronchophony
pectoriloquy
   aphonic p.
   whispered p.
   whispering p.
pectorophony
pediatric
   bronchoscope, p.
   esophagoscope, p.
   feeding tube, p.
   laryngoscope, p.
   nasogastric tube, p.
pedicle
   flap, p.
pedicled
pedicleized
pediodontia
pedistibulum
pedodontia
pedodontics
pedodontist
peenash

PEEP (positive end-expiratory pressure)
Peet nasal rasp
peg tooth
Pelizaeus-Merzbacher disease
pellagra
pellagrin
pellagrous
pellet
   cotton p.
   foil p.
pellicle
   brown p.
   salivary p.
pellicular
pemphigoid
pemphigus
   vulgaris, p.
Pendred disease
pendular nystagmus
pendulous palate
Penn tuning fork
Pennington elevator
Penrose drain
Pentam 300
Pentax bronchoscope
Pentuss
peppermint camphor
peptic esophagitis
per os
perceptive deafness
percuss
percussible
percussion
Perdue tonsillar forceps
perennial
   allergic rhinitis, p.
   allergy, p.
perforation
   Bezold p.
   tooth p.
perforated eardrum
periadenitis
   mucosa necrotica recurrens, p.
perialienitis
periapex
periapical

periapical *(continued)*
   abscess, p.
periauricular
peribronchial
   cuffing, p.
peribronchiolar
peribronchiolitis
peribronchitis
peribulbar
pericapsular
pericemental
   abscess, p.
pericementitis
pericementoclasia
pericementum
perichondritis
perichondrium
periconchal
periconchitis
pericoronal
   abscess, p.
pericoronitis
peridens
peridental
   abscess, p.
peridentitis
peridentium
periesophageal
periesophagitis
perigemmal
periglandular
periglandulitis
periglossitis
periglottic
periglottis
perikyma (pl. perikymata)
perikymata (pl. of perikyma)
perilabyrinth
perilabyrinthitis
perilaryngeal
perilaryngitis
perilymph
perilympha
perilymphadenitis
perilymphangeal
perilymphangitis

perilymphatic
   fistula, p. (PLF)
   labyrinth, p.
perimolysis
perineural fat
periodic
   alternating nystagmus, p. (PAN)
   breathing, p.
periodic breathing
periodontal
   abscess, p.
   anesthesia, p.
   disease, p.
   ligament, p.
   pocket, p.
   probe, p.
periodontia
periodontics
periodontitis
   adult p.
   apical p.
   chronic apical p.
   juvenile p.
   marginal p.
   prepubertal p.
   rapidly progressive p.
   simple p.
   simplex, p.
periodontium
   insertionis, p.
   protectoris, p.
periodontoclasia
periodontology
periodontosis
perioral
periorbital
periosteal
   elevator, p.
periosteotome
periorbital
periosteum
   alveolar p.
   alveolare, p.
periotic
   cartilage, p.
peripharyngeal

peripharyngeal *(continued)*
   space, p.
peripheral
   blood, p.
   cyanosis, p.
   vertigo, p.
periphery
periradicular
perirhinal
perirhizoclasia
perisinuitis
perisinuous
perisinusitis
peristaphyline
perisymphyseal
perisymphysis
perithyroiditis
peritonsillar
   abscess, p.
   tag, p.
peritonsillitis
peritracheal
periuvular
perixenitis
perle
perleche
Per-Lee
   middle ear tube, P.
   myringotomy tube, P.
   ventilating tube, P.
Perlia nucleus
perlingual
permanent
   dentition, p.
   denture, p.
   molar, p.
   teeth, p.
pernasal
peroral
   esophageal prosthesis, p.
peroxide
Peroxyl
perpendicular plate
Pertik diverticulum
pertussis
   immune globulin, p.

pertussis *(continued)*
   -like syndrome, p.
   syndrome, p.
   vaccine, p.
pertussoid
petal-plasty
petechia (pl. petechiae)
petechiae (pl. of petechia)
petechial
   hemorrhage, p.
petiole
petiolus
   epiglottidis, p.
Petrequin ligament
petrolatum gauze
petroleum jelly
petromastoid
   canal, p.
petro-occipital
petropharyngeus
petrosal
   process, p.
   sinus, p.
petrosalpingostaphylinus
petrosectomy
petrositis
petrosomastoid
petrosphenoid
petrosphenoidal
   fissure, p.
   syndrome, p.
petrosquamosal
petrosquamous
   sinus, p.
   suture, p.
petrostaphylinus
petrotympanic
   fissure, p.
petrous
   apex, p.
   artifact, p.
   ganglion, p.
   pyramid, p.
   ridge, p.
Peutz-Jeghers syndrome
Pfau atticus punch

Pfeiffer procedure
Pfeiffer-Grobety technique
PFLAC (pars flaccida portion of tympanic membrane)
phagedenic gingivitis
phantogeusia
phantosmia
pharyngalgia
pharyngeal
   aperture, p.
   aponeurosis, p.
   arches, p.
   bursa, p.
   canal, p.
   cavity, p.
   crisis, p.
   diphtheria, p.
   diverticulum, p.
   flap palatoplasty, p.
   fornix, p.
   function study, p.
   groove, p.
   hemisphincter, p.
   hypophysis, p.
   mirror, p.
   ostium, p.
   pack, p.
   paresis, p.
   plaque, p.
   plexus, p.
   pouch, p.
   recess, p.
   reflex, p.
   septum, p.
   spine, p.
   tonsil, p.
   tube, p.
   wall, p.
   web, p.
pharyngectasia
pharyngectomy
pharyngemphraxis
pharyngeus
pharyngism
pharyngismus
pharyngitic

pharyngitid
pharyngitis
   acute p.
   atrophic p.
   bacterial p.
   catarrhal p.
   chronic p.
   croupous p.
   diphtheritic p.
   follicular p.
   gangrenous p.
   glandular p.
   granular p.
   herpetica, p.
   hypertrophic p.
   keratosa, p.
   membranous p.
   phlegmonous p.
   plague p.
   purulent p.
   sicca, p.
   streptococcal p.
   ulcerosa, p.
   viral p.
pharyngoamygdalitis
pharyngobasilar
pharyngocele
pharyngoconjunctival
   fever, p.
pharyngoceratosis
pharyngoconjunctival
   fever, p.
pharyngoconjunctivitis
pharyngocutaneous
pharyngodynia
pharyngoepiglottic
   arch, p.
   fold, p.
pharyngoepiglottidean
pharyngoesophageal (PE)
   diverticulectomy, p.
   diverticulum, p.
   reconstruction, p.
   sphincter, p.
pharyngoglossal
pharyngoglossus

pharyngogram
pharyngography
pharyngokeratosis
pharyngolaryngeal
   cavity, p.
pharyngolaryngectomy
pharyngolaryngitis
pharyngolith
pharyngology
pharyngolysis
pharyngomaxillary
   space, p.
pharyngomycosis
pharyngonasal
   cavity, p.
pharyngo-oral
   cavity, p.
pharyngopalatine
   arch, p.
pharyngopalatinus
pharyngoparalysis
pharyngopathy
pharyngoperistole
pharyngoplasty
pharyngoplegia
pharyngorhinitis
pharyngorhinoscopy
pharyngorrhagia
pharyngorrhaphy
pharyngorrhea
pharyngosalpingitis
pharyngoscleroma
pharyngoscope
pharyngoscopy
pharyngospasm
pharyngostenosis
pharyngostoma
pharyngostomy
pharyngotherapy
pharyngotome
pharyngotomy
   external p.
   internal p.
   lateral p.
   subhyoid p.
pharyngotonsillitis

pharyngotympanic
   cephalalgia, p.
   tube, p.
pharyngotyphoid
pharyngoxerosis
pharynx
phatnorrhagia
PHC syndrome
phenothiazine
phenozygous
phenylephrine
phenylpropanolamine
Philadelphia
   collar, P.
   tonsil knife, P.
philtrum
   dimple, p.
pHisoHex
phlebectasia
   laryngis, p.
phlegm
phlegmon
   Holz p.
phlegmonous
   laryngitis, p.
   pharyngitis, p.
phoenix abscess
phonal
phonasthenia
phonation
phonatory
   bands, p.
   spasm, p.
phonendoscope
phonetic
   paralysis, p.
phoniatrician
phoniatrics
phonic
phonism
phonogram
phonology
phonomassage
phonometer
phonopathy
phonophobia

phonophotography
phonopsia
phossy
   jaw, p.
   tongue, p.
photic sneezing
photism
photophore
phrenic nerve
phrenoesophageal
phrenoglottic
phthinoid
   bronchitis, p.
physiognomy
physiognosis
physiologic drift
physiological crown
pica
pick
   dental p.
Pickerill imbrication lines
Pickrell zigzag harelip procedure
pickwickian syndrome
picrogeusia
pictorial aphasia
piecrusting
pier
Pierce
   antral trocar, P.
   antral wash tube, P.
   cheek retractor, P.
   double-ended elevator, P.
   mastoid rongeur, P.
   saccade, P.
   submucous dissector, P.
Pierce-O'Connor procedure
pierced ear
Pierre-Robin
   micrognathia, P.
   syndrome, P.
pigmented blue nevus
pillar
   Corti, p. of
   fauces, p. of
   soft palate, p's of
   tonsillar p.

pillar cells
pillar forceps
pillar-grasping forceps
Pilling
   bronchoscope, P.
   duralite tracheal tube, P.
   tracheostomy tube, P.
Pilling bronchoscope
pillow speaker
pilot's vertigo
pin
   endodontic p.
   self-threading p.
Pinaud triangle
pinch graft
pinchcock mechanism
pine tar
ping-pong fracture
pink
   disease, p.
   puffer, p.
   tooth of Mummery, p.
   toothbrush, p.
pinledge
   crown, p.
pinless teeth
pinna
   ear, p. of
   nasi, p.
pinnal
pinpoint cautery
pipe jaw
pirbuterol acetate
piriform
   aperture, p.
   aperture wiring, p.
   fossa, p.
   opening, p.
   process, p.
   sinus, p.
Pirogoff
   angle, P.
   triangle, P.
piston
pit
   auditory p.

176 pit

pit *(continued)*
    basilar p.
    oblong p. of arytenoid cartilage
    olfactory p.
    nasal p.
    pterygoid p.
    triangular p. of arytenoid cartilage
pit caries
pit cavity
pit and fissure sealant
Pitt Speaking Tracheostomy Tube
pituitary forceps
PL (pulpolingual)
PLA (pulpolabial or pulpolinguoaxial)
plague
    pharyngeal p.
    pharyngitis, p.
Plak-Vac
plana (pl. of planum)
plane
    Aeby p.
    alveolocondylar p.
    axiolabiolingual p.
    axiomesiodistal p.
    Baer p.
    bite p.
    Daubenton p.
    Frankfort horizontal p.
    frontal p.
    Meckel p.
    occlusal p.
planing
    root p.
plantation
planum (pl. plana)
    nuchal p.
    occipital p.
    orbital p.
    temporal p.
plaque
    dental p.
plasmacytoma
plaster
    head cap, p.
    mustard p.
    Paris, p. of

plastic
    bronchitis, p.
    mouth guard, p.
    surgery, p.
Plasti-Pore
plate
    alar p.
    auditory p.
    bite p.
    clinoid p.
    cortical p.
    cough p.
    cribriform p.
    dental p.
    die p.
    foot p.
    frontal p.
    frontonasal p.
    horizontal p. of palatine bone
    jumping the bite p.
    Kingsley p.
    lingual p.
    oral p.
    orbital p. of ethmoid bone
    palatal p.
    palate p.
    paper p.
    parietal p.
    perpendicular p. of ethmoid bone
    perpendicular p. of palatine bone
    pharyngeal p.
    pterygoid p.
    Sherman p.
    spring p.
    tympanic p.
    vertical p. of palatine bone
    wing p.
plateau of speech
plated die
platinectomy
platinosis
platinum foil
platyglossal
platyrrhine
platysma
platysmal

platysmaplasty
platystaphyline
platystencephaly
Plaut angina
Plaut-Vincent angina
plectrum
pledget
plegaphonia
pleomorphic adenoma
pleonotia
pleurisy
pleuritic
pleurobronchitis
pleurodont
pleuroesophageal
plexus
  carotid p.
  cavernous p.
  dental p.
  esophageal p.
  infraorbital p.
  internal carotid p.
  Kiesselbach p.
  laryngeal p.
  parotid p.
  pharyngeal p.
  pterygoid p.
  Raschkow, p. of
  tonsillar p.
  tympanic p.
PLF (perilymphatic fistula)
plica (pl. plicae)
  epiglottic p.
  lacrimal p.
  nasi, p.
  nervi laryngei, p.
  salpingopharyngea, p.
  stapedis, p.
  sublingualis, p.
  supratonsillaris, p.
  triangularis, p.
  vocalis, p.
plicadentin
plicae (pl. of plica)
plicated tongue
plicotomy

pliers
plug
plugged
  ears, p.
  nose, p.
plugger
  automatic p.
  back-action p.
  foot p.
Plummer
  bougie, P.
  water-filled pneumatic esophageal
    dilator, P.
Plummer-Vinson syndrome
plumper
plunging goiter
PM (pulpomesial)
PND (paroxysmal nocturnal dyspnea or
  postnasal drainage or postnasal drip)
pneumatic
  bag esophageal dilatation, p.
  otoscope, p.
pneumatization
pneumatized
pneumato-otoscope
pneumato-otoscopy
pneumoalveolography
pneumomediastinum
pneumothorax
pneumotympanum
pnigophobia
PO (by mouth)
pocket
  complex p.
  compound p.
  gingival p.
  infrabony p.
  intra-alveolar p.
  intrabony p.
  periodontal p.
  pseudo-p.
  pus p.
  relative p.
  Seessel p.
  simple p.
  subcrestal p.

pocket *(continued)*
   suprabony p.
   supracrestal p.
pocket probe
pogonion
point
   angle, p.
   Ar, p.
   angle, p.
   auricular p.
   Bo, p.
   Broca p.
   craniometric p.
   deaf p's of ear
   gutta-percha p.
   jugal p.
   lacrimal p.
   malar p.
   median mandibular p.
   mental p.
   metopic p.
   nasal p.
   preauricular p.
   R, p.
   SE, p.
   SO, p.
   spinal p.
   subnasal p.
   supra-auricular p.
   supranasal p.
   supraorbital p.
point tenderness
Poirier
   glands, P.
   line, P.
poker facies
polio laryngoscope
polishing brush
Politzer
   angular ear knife, P.
   bag, P.
   ear perforator, P.
   otoscope, P.
   speculum, P.
   test, P.
   treatment, P.

politzerization
Polk finger goniometer
pollen
   allergy, p.
   asthma, p.
pollenogenic
pollinosis
polly-beak nose
poltophagy
polyadenitis
polyadenopathy
polycarboxylate cement
polychondritis
polycythemia
polydentia
polyethylene
   collar button, p.
   plate, p.
   prosthesis, p.
   tube, p.
polygactin
polyinfection
polymethyl methacrylate
polymyxin
polyodontia
polyotia
polyp
   antrochoanal p.
   choanal p.
   gum p.
   Hopmann p.
   larynx, p's of
   nasal p's
polypectomy
polypoid
polyphyodont dentition
polyposis
polysialia
polysilaxane
polysinusectomy
polysinuitis
polysinusitis
polysomnography
polystomatous
polytef
polytetrafluoroethylene (PTFE)

polytomography
polyurethrane foam embolus
polyvalent allergy
pomum adami (Adam's apple)
pond fracture
pontic
ponticular
ponticulus
    auriculae, p.
    promontorii, p.
pooling of saliva
Pope
    Merocel ear packing, P.
    Merocel ear wick, P.
popliteal
    -pterygium syndrome, p.
    web syndrome, p.
Poppers tonsillar guillotine
porcelain
    dental p.
porcelain crown
porcelain filling
porcelain jacket
porcelain laminate
porcelain veneer
porcelaneous
porcelanous
Porex facial implant
porion
Porites coral
PORP (partial ossicular reconstructive or replacement prosthesis)
Porta-Stat
portepolisher
Porter sign
Portex
    speaking tube, P.
    tracheostomy tube, P.
Portmann interposition procedure
porus
    acusticus externus, p.
    acusticus externus osseus, p.
    acusticus internus, p.
    acusticus internus osseus, p.
    gustatorius, p.
positional

positional *(continued)*
    nystagmus, p.
    vertigo, p.
positioner
    tooth p.
positive
    end-expiratory pressure, p. (PEEP)
    fistula test, p.
postaural
    approach, p.
    arches, p.
postaurale
postauricular
    approach, p.
    arterial flap, p.
    incision, p.
postcanine
postconcussional syndrome
postdam area
posterior
    cricoarytenoid cartilage, p.
    facial height, p.
    fossa, p.
    fossa myelography, p.
    fossa tumor, p.
    nasal spine, p.
    pack, p.
    palatal seal area, p.
    palate hook, p.
    pillar, p.
    ramal plane, p.
    triangle, p.
posteroclusion
posterula
posthyoid
posthyperventilation
    apnea, p.
    syndrome, p.
postlingual
    deafness, p.
postmastoid
postnares
postnarial
postnasal
    balloon, p.
    catarrh, p.

postnasal *(continued)*
   discharge, p.
   drainage, p. (PND)
   dressing, p.
   drip, p. (PND)
   tube, p.
postpalatine
postprandial
postsphenoid
posttracheostomy
posttussis
posttussive
   suction, p.
postural
   drainage and percussion, p. (PD&P)
   vertigo, p.
posturography
potential acuity meter (PAM)
Pott's puffy tumor
Potter
   facies, P.
   syndrome, P.
   tonsillar forceps
potters' asthma
pouch
   anterior p. of Troltsch
   branchial p.
   craniobuccal p.
   craniopharyngeal p.
   laryngeal p.
   neurobuccal p.
   pharyngeal p.
   posterior p. of Troltsch
   Prussak p.
   Rathke p.
   Seessel p.
   visceral p.
pouched
pouching
poultice
pouting
practolol
prandial
Pratt
   antrum curette, P.
   ethmoid curette, P.

Pratt *(continued)*
   hook, P.
   nasal curette, P.
preaurale
preauricular
prebase
precementum
precision anchorage
precocious dentition
predeciduous dentition
predentin
preepiglottic
preextraction cast
preferential anosmia
prefrontal
   bone of von Bardeleben, p.
preglottic
   tonsillitis, p.
pregnancy gingivitis
pregonium
prehyoid
prelacrimal abscess
prelaryngeal
   lymph nodes, p.
prelingual deafness
premature contact
premaxilla
premaxillary palate
premolar
prenares
prenasale
preoperative cast
preoral
   gut, p.
prepalatal
preparation
   biomechanical p.
   cavity p.
prepared cavity
preprandial
presbyacusia
presbycusis
presbyesophagus
presphenoid
pressure point
pressured speech

prethyroideal
prethyroidean
pretracheal
   fascia, p.
   lymph node, p.
   space, p.
preventive dentistry
prevertebral
   fascia, p.
   space, p.
prevertiginous
prevesical
   facial cleft, p.
   space, p.
Preyer reflex
Price-Thomas bronchial forceps
primary
   dentition, p.
   fistula, p.
   teeth, p.
Primatene Mist
primordial cyst
Prince tonsillar scissors
Prince-Potts tonsillar scissors
prism
prisma (pl. prismata)
prismata (pl. of prisma)
   adamantina, p.
privet cough
prizefighter ear
probang
probe
   dental p.
   lacrimal p.
   periodontal p.
   pocket p.
   root canal p.
process
   alar p.
   alveolar p.
   basilar p.
   Blumenbach, p. of
   clinoid p.
   condyloid p.
   coronoid p.
   ethmoid p.

process *(continued)*
   Folius, p. of
   frontal p.
   frontonasal p.
   frontosphenoidal p.
   hamular p.
   infraorbital p.
   jugular p.
   lacrimal p.
   lenticular p.
   malar p.
   mandibular p.
   mastoid p.
   maxillary p.
   nasal p.
   odontoblastic p.
   odontoid p.
   orbital p.
   palatine p.
   postglenoid p.
   pterygoid p.
   styloid p.
   Soemmering, p. of
   Tomes p.
   uncinate p. of ethmoid bone
   vocal p.
   zygomatic p.
   zygomatico-orbital p. of maxilla
processus
procheilon
Proctor
   elevator, P.
   retractor, P.
productive
   bronchitis, p.
   cough, p.
   phlegm, p.
   sputum, p.
Proetz
   displacement, P.
   mouth gag, P.
   tongue depressor, P.
   treatment, P.
Proetz-Jansen mouth gag
profile
   analysis, p.

profile *(continued)*
   line, p.
proglossis
proglottid
progonoma
prognathia
prognathic
prognathism
prognathometer
prognathous
projecting jaw
projection
prolabium
prominence
prominentia (pl. prominentiae)
   canalis facialis, p.
   canalis semicircularis lateralis, p.
   laryngea, p.
   mallearis membranae tympani, p.
   malleolaris membranae tympani, p.
   spiralis, p.
   styloidea, p.
prominentiae (pl. of prominentia)
promontoria (pl. of promontorium)
promontorium (pl. promontoria)
   faciei, p.
   tympani, p.
promontory
   tympanic cavity, p. of
prong
pro-otic
Propadrine
propalinal
prophylactic
prophylaxis
   dental p.
   oral p.
Proplast
   facial implant, P.
   chin implant, P.
   -HA hydroxyapatite, P.
   nasal implant, P.
   -Teflon implant, P.
propons
proptosis
prosopalgia

prosopantritis
prosopectasia
prosopoanoschisis
prosopodiplegia
prosopodynia
prosopodysmorphia
prosoponeuralgia
prosopoplegia
prosoposchisis
prosopospasm
prosopus varus
prostheses (pl. of prosthesis)
prosthesis (pl. prostheses)
   antireflux p.
   cleft palate p.
   dental p.
   maxillofacial p.
   speech-aid p.
prosthetic
   appliance, p.
   dentistry, p.
   device, p.
   joint implant, p.
prosthetics
   dental p.
   denture p.
   facial p.
   maxillofacial p.
prosthetist
prosthion
prosthodontics
prosthodontist
proteolysis-chelation theory
proteolytic theory
protocone
protoconid
Protoplast
protraction
   mandibular p.
   maxillary p.
protrude
protrusion
   bimaxillary p.
   bimaxillary dentoalveolar p.
protrusive
   occlusion, p.

protuberance
  chin, p. of
  laryngeal p.
  mental p.
  palatine p.
  teeth, p. of
protuberant
  jaw, p.
  teeth, p.
protuberantia
  mentalis, p.
Proventil
  inhaler, P.
  Repetabs, P.
provisional denture
proximal contact
proximate contact
proximobuccal
proximolabial
proximolingual
prune juice sputum
Prussak
  fibers, P.
  pouch, P.
  space, P.
psalterial cord
psellism
pseudoacousis
pseudoacousma
pseudoalveolar
pseudoanodontia
pseudobronchiectasis
pseudochancre
pseudocholesteatoma
pseudocroup
pseudoephedrine
pseudogeusesthesia
pseudogeusia
pseudoglottic
pseudoglottis
pseudohypoparathyroidism
pseudomembranous
  bronchitis, p.
  croup, p.
pseudomonal
Pseudomonas

Pseudomonas *(continued)*
  aeruginosa, P.
pseudonystagmus
pseudoptyalism
pseudosmia
pseudostratified
pseudotrismus
pseudovoice
psi (pounds per square inch)
psittacosis
psomophagia
psychauditory
psychic deafness
psychoauditory
psychogeusic
psycholinguistics
psychosensory aphasia
ptarmic
ptarmus
pterion
pterygium
  colli, p.
pterygoid
  apophysis, p.
  canal, p.
  fissure, p.
  fossa, p.
  hamulus, p.
  notch, p.
  pit, p.
  plate, p.
  plexus, p.
  process, p.
  stripper, p.
  tubercle, p.
pterygoideus
  internus, p.
  lateralis, p.
  medialis, p.
pterygomandibular
  ligament, p.
  raphe, p.
pterygomaxillary
  fissure, p.
pterygopalatine
  canal, p.

pterygopalatine *(continued)*
   fossa, p.
   groove, p.
PTFE (polytetrafluoroethylene)
ptosis
   -epicanthus syndrome, p.
ptotic
ptyalagogue
ptyalectasis
ptyalin
ptyalism
ptyalith
ptyalize
ptyalocele
ptyalogenic
ptyalogogue
ptyalography
ptyalolith
ptyalolithiasis
ptyalolithotomy
ptyaloreaction
ptyalorrhea
ptysis
pug nose
Pulmo-Aid nebulizer
pulmonary cough
pulp
   coronal p.
   dead p.
   dental p.
   devitalized p.
   enamel p.
   exposed p.
   necrotic p.
   nonvital p.
   putrescent p.
   radicular p.
   tooth p.
   vital p.
pulpa (pl. pulpae)
   coronale, p.
   dentis, p.
   radicularis, p.
pulp abscess
pulpaceous
pulpae (pl. of pulpa)

pulpal (P)
   abscess, p.
pulpalgia
pulp amputation
pulp calcification
pulp canal
pulp capping
pulp cavity
pulpectomy
pulpefaction
pulp exposure
pulp extirpation
pulpiform
pulpitides (pl. of pulpitis)
   anachoretic p.
   closed p.
   hyperplastic p.
   open p.
pulpless
pulpoaxial (PA)
pulpobuccal (PB)
pulpobuccoaxial (PBA)
pulpodistal (PD)
pulpodontics
pulpolabial (PLA)
pulpolingual (PL)
pulpolinguoaxial (PLA)
pulpomesial (PM)
pulpotomy
pulp stone
pulp vitality
pulpy
pump
   dental p.
pumper
pumping
punch
   adenoid p.
   tonsil p.
punched-out
punctate lesion
punctum
punctumeter
pure tone audiometry
Puritan Bubble-Jet
pursed-lip breathing

purulence
purulent
　drainage, p.
　exudate, p.
　otitis media, p.
pus
　pocket, p.
push-back palatoplasty
pustular
　pharyngitis, p.
　tonsillitis, p.
pustule
pusy drainage
putrefaction
putrified
putrify
putrescent
　pulp, p.
　pulpitis, p.
putrid
　bronchitis, p.
Putterman concaved clamp
pyemia
pyemic
pyknophrasia
pyknosis
Pynchon
　applicator, P.
　mouth gag, P.
　nasal speculum, P.
　tongue depressor, P.
Pynchon-Lillie tongue depressor
pyoblennorrhea

pyocele
pyogenic
　granuloma, p.
pyolabyrinthitis
pyophagia
pyoptysis
pyorrhea
　alveolaris, p.
　Schmutz p.
pyorrheal
pyostatic
pyostomatitis
　vegetans, p.
pyramid
　Lalouette p.
　light, p. of
　olfactory p.
　petrous p.
　temporal bone, p. of
　thyroid, p. of
　tympanum, p. of
　vestibule, p. of
　Wistar p's
pyramidal
　cartilage, p.
　eminence, p.
pyramidalis
　auriculae, p.
pyramidotomy
pyramis
pyriform
　aperture, p.
　aperture wiring, p.

Additional entries

Q

Q-tip
quadrangle
quadrangular
   membrane, q.
quadrant
   dental q.
quadrantal cephalalgia
quadricuspid
quadrilateral
   cartilage, q.
   plate, q.
quartz
Quatrefage angle
Queckenstedt test
quick-cure resin

quiet breath sounds
quilted sutures
Quimby gum scissors
quinine sulfate
quinquecuspid
quinsy
   lingual q.
quinsy sore throat
Quint
   J-R Unit, Q.
   Sectograph, Q.
Quinton suction biopsy instrument
Quire mechanical finger forceps
Quisling hammer

Additional entries

R

rabbit nose
rabid
rabies
    dumb r.
    furious r.
    paralytic r.
rabiform
raccoon eyes
racemose adenoma
rad (radiation absorbed dose)
radiation
    absorbed dose, r. (rad)
    caries, r.
    gingivitis, r.
    stomatitis, r.
radical neck dissection (RND)
radices (pl. of radix)
radicular cyst
radiectomy
radioactive
    iodine, r. (RAI)
    iodine uptake, r. (RAIU)
radioallergosorbent test (RAST)
radiodontics
radiograph
    bitewing r.
    cephalometric r.
    dental r.
    lateral cephalometric r.
    lateral ramus r.
    lateral skull r.
    maxillary sinus r.
    panoramic r.
    Panorex r.
    periapical r.
    submental r.
    Towne projection r.
    Waters view r.
radiographic-evident sponge
radiography
radiolucent bite block
radionuclide imaging
radiopaque

radiosialographic
radisectomy
radix (pl. radices)
Radovan tissue expander
RAE endotracheal tube
rag wheel
Ragnell
    operation, R.
    scissors, R.
ragweed
RAI (radioactive iodine)
railroad nystagmus
RAIU (radioactive iodine uptake)
Raimondi scalp hemostatic forceps
rake teeth
rales
Ralks
    ear knife, R.
    elevator, R.
    tuning fork, r.
Ralks-Davis mouth gag
Ramadier intrapetrosal drainage
Rambo musculoplasty
Ramfjord index
rami (pl. of ramus)
Ramitec
rampant caries
rampart
Ramsay Hunt syndrome
ramus (pl. rami)
    alveolar r.
    bronchial r.
    mandibular r.
Randall procedure
random flap
ranine
Ranke angle
ranula
ranular
raphe
    buccal r.
    palate, r. of
    palatine r.

raphe *(continued)*
    palpebral r.
    pharyngeal r.
    pharyngis, r.
    pharynx, r. of
    pterygomandibular r.
    tongue, r. of
Rappaport classification
Raschkow plexus
rash
    butterfly r.
    gum r.
    heat r.
    maculopapular r.
    red r.
    tooth r.
    wandering r.
Rasmussen nerve fibers
rasp
raspatory
rasped
raspberry tongue
RAST (radioallergosorbent test)
Rathe
    pocket, R.
    pouch, R.
    tumor, R.
Rau
    apophysis, R.
    process, R.
ravian process
Ray nasal speculum
Ray-Parsons-Sunday staphlorrhaphy elevator
RDF (rotary door flap)
RDS (respiratory distress syndrome)
Read oral curette
reamer
reattachment
rebase
rebreathing mask
recanalization
receding
    chin, r.
    gums, r.
    jaw, r.

receptive aphasia
recess
    azygoesophageal r.
    cochlear r.
    epitympanic r. (EPR)
    Hyrtl r.
    infundibular r.
    infundibuliform r.
    internal ear r.
    lacrimal r.
    laryngopharyngeal r.
    nasopalatine r.
    nasopharynx, r. of
    pharyngeal r.
    piriform r.
    Reichert r.
    Rosenmuller, r. of
    sphenoethmoidal r.
    spherical r.
    supratonsillar r.
    Troltsch, r. of
    tympanic membrane r.
    vestibule, r. of
recession
    gingival r.
    gum r.
recessus
    cochlearis vestibuli, r.
    ellipticus vestibuli, r.
    epitympanicus, r.
    membranae tympani anterior, r.
    membranae tympani posterior, r.
    membranae tympani superior, r.
    pharyngeus, r.
    piriformis, r.
    pro utriculo, r.
    sphenoethmoidalis, r.
    sphenoethmoidalis osseus, r.
    sphericus vestibuli, r.
reciprocal
    anchorage, r.
    arm, r.
    force, r.
reciprocating saw
reciprocation
recontour

record
    centric interocclusal r.
    face-bow r.
    functional chew-in r.
    interocclusal r.
    jaw relation r.
    lateral interocclusal r.
    maxillomandibular r.
    occluding centric relation r.
    profile r.
    protrusive r.
    terminal jaw relation r.
    protrusive interocclusal r.
recruitment
recurrent laryngeal nerve
red
    gum, r.
    Robinson catheter, r.
    rubber catheter, r.
    strawberry tongue, r.
Reese
    dermatome, R.
    technique, R.
reflex
    asthma, r.
    cough, r.
reflux
    esophageal r.
    gastroesophageal r.
reflux esophagitis
    classification of r.
        E-I   (erythema, edema)
        E-II (erosions)
        E-III (localized deformity)
        E-IV (stricture)
refractory
    cast, r.
    flask, r.
Refsum disease
regainer
    -maintainer, r.
Regaud tumor
regional lymph nodes
registration
    maxillomandibular r.
Reglan

Regnoli operation
regurgitate
regurgitation
Reichert
    cartilage, R.
    recess, R.
Reichert/Meindinger (R/M) stereotactic system
Reid base line
reimplantation
Reiner-Beck tonsil snare
Reiner-Knight ethmoid-cutting forceps
reinforced anchorage
Reissner membrane
relation
    jaw r.
    acentric r.
    acquired acentric jaw r.
    buccolingual r.
    centric jaw r.
    eccentric jaw r.
    jaw r.
    lateral occlusal r.
    maxillomandibular r.
    median jaw r.
    median retruded jaw r.
    occlusal jaw r.
    posterior border jaw r.
    protrusive jaw r.
    rest jaw r.
    ridge r.
    unstrained jaw r.
relaxed skin tension lines (RSTL)
relaxing incision
relief
    area, r.
    chamber, r.
reline
rem (roentgen-equivalent-man)
remodeling
    temporomandibular joint r.
reparative dentin
replant
replantation
repositioning
    jaw r.

resection
  window r.
reserve cells
residual dental arch
resilient nystagmus
resin
  acrylic r.
  activated r.
  autopolymer r.
  cold-curing r.
  composite r.
  copolymer r.
  direct filling r.
  epoxy r.
  heat-curing r.
  quick-cure r.
  self-curing r.
  styrene r.
resin cement
resorption
  lacunae, r.
respirator
  -dependent, r.
  mask, r.
respiratory
  acidosis, r.
  alkalosis, r.
  anemometer, r.
  apparatus, r.
  arrest, r.
  center, r.
  compromise, r.
  distress syndrome, r. (RDS)
  embarrassment, r.
  excursion, r.
  failure, r.
  insufficiency, r.
  mucosa, r.
  quotient, r.
  sounds, r.
  standstill, r.
  stridor, r.
  support, r.
  syncytial virus, r. (RSV)
  tract, r.
  upper r. infection (URI)

respirometer
rest
  incisal r.
  lingual r.
  Malassez r.
  occlusal r.
  precision r.
  recessed r.
  semiprecision r.
  surface r.
rest area
rest jaw relation
rest seat
restbite
restoration
  buccal r.
  dental r.
  facial r.
  prosthetic r.
  temporary r.
restorative
resuscitate
resuscitation
resuscitator
retained root
retainer
  continuous bar r.
  direct r.
  Hawley r.
  indirect r.
  matrix r.
  space r.
retainer arch bar
retarded dentition
retch
retention
  lug, r.
Rethi
  incision, R.
  nasal tip reconstruction, R.
  rhinoplasty, R.
reticulosis
  polymorphic r.
retraction nystagmus
retrenchment
retroauricular

retroauricular *(continued)*
  incision, r.
  sulcus, r.
retrobronchial
retrobuccal
retrobulbar
  neuritis, r.
retrocochlear
retrocollic
  spasm, r.
retrocollis
retrodental
retroesophageal
retrofacial
  cells of Broca, r.
retrofill
retrofilling
retrognathia
retrognathic
retrognathism
retrograde amalgam filling
retrohyoid bursa
retrolabyrinthine
retrolingual
retromandibular
retromastoid
retromolar
  fossa, r.
  pad, r.
  trigone, r.
retronasal
retro-ocular
retroparotid
retropharyngeal
  abscess, r.
  lymph nodes, r.
  space, r.
retropharyngitis
retropharynx
retrosinus
retrotonsillar
  abscess, r.
retrotracheal
retrovirus
retro-ocular
retrude

retruded tooth
retrusion
retrusive
Retzius
  lines of R.
  parallel striae, R.
Reuter
  bobbin tube, R.
  collar-button tube, R.
  stainless steel bobbin, R.
reverberation
Reverdin
  graft, R.
  needle, R.
reverse
  Gillies for trimalar procedure, r.
  -L osteotomy, r.
reversible obstructive airway disease
Reyer test
rhabdomyolysis
rhabdomyosarcoma
rhaebocrania
rhagades
rhagadiform
Rhese position for paranasal sinuses
rheum
rheumic
rhinal
  fissure, r.
  sulcus, r.
rhinalgia
rhinallergosis
rhinedema
rhinencephalocele
rhinencephalon
rhinencephalus
rhinenchysis
rhinesthesia
rhineurynter
rhinion
rhinism
rhinitis
  acute catarrhal r.
  allergic r.
  anaphylactic r.
  atrophic r.

rhinitis *(continued)*
   caseosa, r.
   catarrhal r.
   chronic hyperplastic r.
   chronic hypertrophic r.
   croupous r.
   dyscrinic r.
   fibrinous r.
   gangrenous r.
   hypertrophic r.
   infectious r.
   influenzal r.
   membranous r.
   nonairflow r.
   nonseasonal allergic r.
   perennial r.
   periodic r.
   pseudomembranous r.
   purulent r.
   scrofulous r.
   sicca, r.
   suppurative r.
   syphilitic r.
   tuberculous r.
   vasomotor r.
rhinoanemometer
rhinoantritis
rhinobyon
rhinocanthectomy
rhinocele
rhinocephalia
rhinocephalus
rhinocephaly
rhinocheiloplasty
rhinocleisis
rhinocoele
rhinodacryolith
rhinodynia
rhinoentomophthoromycosis
Rhinoestrus
   purpureus, R.
rhinogenous
rhinokyphectomy
rhinokyphosis
rhinolalia
   aperta, r.

rhinolalia *(continued)*
   clausa, r.
   open r.
rhinolaryngitis
rhinolaryngology
rhinolaryngoscope
rhinolaryngoscopy
rhinolith
rhinolithiasis
rhinologist
rhinology
rhinomanometer
rhinomanometry
rhinometer
rhinomiosis
rhinommectomy
rhinomycosis
rhinonasopharyngitis
rhinonecrosis
rhinonemmeter
rhinoneurosis
rhinopathia
   vasomotoria, r.
rhinopathy
rhinopharyngeal
rhinopharyngitis
   mutilans, r.
rhinopharyngocele
rhinopharyngolith
rhinopharynx
rhinophonia
rhinophore
rhinophycomycosis
rhinophyma
rhinoplastic
rhinoplasty
   Carpue r.
   dactylocostal r.
   English r.
   Indian r.
   Italian r.
   Joseph r.
   tagliacotian r.
rhinoplasty implant
rhinoplasty saw
rhinoplasty scissors

ridge 193

rhinopneumonitis
rhinopolypus
rhinoreaction
Rhino Rocket injector
rhinorrhagia
rhinorrhaphy
rhinorrhea
  cerebrospinal r.
  green r.
  gustatory r.
rhinosalpingitis
rhinoscleroma
rhinoscope
rhinoscopic
  mirror, r.
rhinoscopy
  anterior r.
  posterior r.
rhinoseptoplasty
rhinosinusitis
Rhinosporidium
  seeberi, R.
rhinosporidiosis
rhinostegnosis
rhinostenosis
rhinostomy
rhinotomy
rhinotracheitis
rhinovaccination
rhinoviral
rhinovirus
rhitidectomy
rhitodosis
rhizodontropy
rhizodontrypy
rhizoid
Rhizopus
  nigricans, R.
rhizotomy
rhombic lip
rhomboid
rhonchal
rhonchi (pl. of rhonchus)
rhonchial
rhonchorous cough
rhonchus (pl. rhonchi)

Rhoton microsurgical forceps
rhythmic nystagmus
rhytidectomy
rhytidoplasty
rhytidosis
ribbon
  arch, r.
  arch appliance, r.
  muscles, r.
Ribes ganglion
Richards
  mastoid ethmoid curette, R.
  tonsil-seizing forceps, R.
Richardson right-angle ear knife
Richmond crown
rickets
Ricketts law
rickettsial
rictal
rictus
Ridell operation
riders' vertigo
ridge
  alveolar r.
  buccocervical r.
  buccogingival r.
  carotid r.
  dental r.
  edentulous r.
  linguocervical r.
  linguogingival r.
  longitudinal r. of hard palate
  mandibular neck, r. of
  mylohyoid r.
  nose, r. of
  oblique r.
  palatine r's
  Passavant r.
  petrous r.
  pharyngeal r.
  pterygoid r.
  residual r.
  sphenoid r.
  sublingual r.
  supplemental r.
  supracondylar r.

ridge *(continued)*
    supraorbital r.
    taste r's
ridge reduction
ridge relation
ridging
Ridley sinus
Ridpath ethmoid curette
Ridson wiring
Riecker respiration bronchoscope
Riedel thyroiditis
Riga-Fede disease
Riggs disease
rigid
    bronchoscope, r.
    bronchoscopy, r.
    esophagoscope, r.
    esophagoscopy, r.
rim
    bite r.
    occlusion r.
rim fracture
rim incision
rim strip technique
rima (pl. rimae)
    glottidis, r.
    glottidis cartilaginea, r.
    glottidis membranacea, r.
    intercartilaginous r.
    intermembranous r.
    mouth, r. of
    oris, r.
    vestibuli, r.
    vocalis, r.
rimae (pl. of rima)
rimal
ring
    Schatzki r.
    tracheal r.
    tympanic r.
ring curette
ring fracture
Ringer's
    lactate, R.
    solution, R.
ringing in the ears

Rinne test
Riolan
    bones, R.
    bouquet, R.
    nosegay, R.
    ossicles, R.
Risdon
    approach, R.
    extraoral incision, R.
risorius
risus
    caninus, r.
    sardonicus, r.
rivinian
    notch, r.
    segment, r.
Rivinus
    canals, R.
    ducts, R.
    foramen, R.
    gland, R.
    incisure, R.
    ligament, R.
    membrane, R.
    notch, R.
rivus lacrimalis
RM (Reichert/Meindinger) stereotactic system
RND (radical neck dissection)
Robb tonsillar forceps
Roberts
    applicator, R.
    bronchial forceps, R.
    esophagoscope, R.
    laryngoscope, R.
    nasal snare, R.
    operation, R.
Robertshaw double-lumen endotracheal tube
Robertson
    forceps, R.
    knife, R.
Robin syndrome
Robinow syndrome
Robinson
    catheter, R.

Robinson *(continued)*
    stapedectomy, R.
    tonsillar suction, R.
Robitussin
Rockey trachea cannula
Rockwell hardness test
rod
    Corti r's
    enamel r's
    House r.
    olfactory r.
Roeder treatment
Roger
    reflex, R.
    syndrome, R.
Roger Anderson
    facial fracture appliance, R.
    pin fixation, R.
Rogers dissector
Rokitansky diverticulum
Rokitansky-Cushing ulcers
Roller nucleus
rolling hernia
Romadier procedure
Roman nose
Romberg
    disease, R.
    facial deformity, R.
Ronne nasal step
Ronneau retractor
Ronnis
    adenoid punch, R.
    cutting forceps, R.
roof of mouth
root
    anatomical r.
    cochlear r. of vestibulocochlear nerve
    facial r.
    intermediate r. of olfactory trigone
    lingual r.
    motor r's of submandibular ganglion
    motor r. of trigeminal nerve
    nasociliary r. of ciliary ganglion
    nose, r. of
    olfactory r.
    palatine r.

root *(continued)*
    retained r.
    tongue, r. of
    tooth, r. of
    vestibular r. of vestibulocochlear nerve
root abscess
root amputation
root ankylosis
root canal
    broach, r.
    cement, r.
    dehiscence, r.
    filling, r.
    probe, r.
    spreader, r.
root elevator
root-end amputation
root-end filling
root-end resection
root pick
root planing
root resection
root resorption
root sheath
rooting reflex
rootless teeth
ropy saliva
rosary-bead esophagus
rose cold
Rose
    cleft lip repair, R.
    L-type nose bridge prosthesis, R.
    position, R.
    procedure, R.
    tamponade, R.
    tracheal retractor, R.
Rosen
    ear probe, R.
    endaural probe, R.
    explorer, R.
    fenestrator, R.
    knife, R.
    needle, R.
    operation, R.
    pick, R.
    probe, R.

Rosen *(continued)*
    separator, R.
    stapes mobilization, R.
    tube, R.
Rosenmuller
    cavity, R.
    fossa, R.
Rosenthal canal
roseola
Roser mouth gag
Roser-Thompson cleft lip repair
rosin
Rostan asthma
rostriform
rostrum
    sinus, r. of
    sphenoidal r.
rotary
    door flap, r. (RDF)
    nystagmus, r.
    vertigo, r.
rotation
    advancement flap repair, r.
    flap, r.
    test, r.
    tooth, r. of
rotational chair
rotatory
    spasm, r.
    vertigo, r.
Rothmund-Thompson syndrome
rouge
Rouge operation
round window
Rowland
    nasal hump forceps, r.
    osteotome, R.

Rowland *(continued)*
    rongeur, R.
Royce perforator
RSTL (relaxed skin tension lines)
RSV (respiratory syncytial virus)
rubber dam
    punch, r.
rubella
rubeola
rubiginous
Rubin
    cartilage planer, R.
    septal morselizer, R.
    tube, R.
Rubinstein syndrome
Rubinstein-Taybi syndrome
ruga (pl. rugae)
    palatina, r.
rugae (pl. of ruga)
rugose
running W-plasty
rupture
    bronchial r.
    esophageal r.
    orbicularis oris, r. of
    tracheobronchial r.
ruptured
    esophagus, r.
    tracheobronchial tree, r.
Rusch
    laryngoscope, R.
Ruskin
    antral needle, R.
    forceps, R.
    mastoid rongeur, R.
Ruysch tube
Ryle tube

Additional entries

S

saber-sheath trachea
sac
    dental s.
    enamel s.
    Hilton s.
    lacrimal s.
    laryngeal s.
sacciform
saccular
    bronchiectasis, s.
sacculated
sacculation
sacculation
saccule
    ear, s. of
    laryngeal s.
    larynx, s. of
    vestibule, s. of
sacculi (pl. of sacculus)
sacculocochlear
    canal, s.
sacculoutricular
    canal, s.
    duct, s.
sacculus (pl. sacculi)
    communis, s.
    dentis, s.
    lacrimalis, s.
    laryngis, s.
    morgagnii, s.
    proprius, s.
    rotundus, s.
    sphaericus, s.
    ventricularis, s.
    vestibularis, s.
saddle
    denture base s.
saddle area
saddle-back nose
saddle connector
saddle nose
Saethre-Chotzen syndrome
Safar

Safar *(continued)*
    bronchoscope, S.
    -S airway, S.
Safian tip rhinoplasty
Sage
    snare, S.
    tonsil snare, S.
Sage-Clark cheilectomy
sagging jowls
sagittal
    sinus, s.
    -split osteotomy, s.
    splitting of mandible, s.
    suture, s.
St. Clair-Thompson
    adenotome, S.
    curette, S.
Sajou laryngeal forceps
salaam spasm
salabrasion
Salem nasogastric tube
saline
    gargle, s.
    irrigation, s.
    lavage, s.
    spray, s.
Salinger nasal reducer
saliva
    artificial s.
    chorda s.
    ganglionic s.
    lingual s.
    parotid s.
    ropy s.
    sublingual s.
    submaxillary s.
    sympathetic s.
salivant
salivary
    calculus, s.
    corpuscle, s.
    digestion, s.
    duct, s.

salivary *(continued)*
   fistula, s.
   gland, s.
   gland capsule, s.
   gland scan, s.
   gland tumor, s.
   gland virus, s. (SGV)
   parotid gland, s.
   stone, s.
   sublingual gland, s.
   submaxillary gland, s.
   tubes, s.
   view, s.
salivate
salivation
salivator
salivatory
salmon patch
salpingitis
   eustachian s.
salpingocatheterism
salpingopalatine
salpingopharyngeal
   fold, s.
   muscle, s.
salpingoscope
salpingoscopy
salpingostaphyline
salpingostenochoria
salpinx
   auditiva, s.
salt water gargle
Salter line
salute
   allergic s.
saluting
salvarsan throat irrigation tube
Salvatore-Maloney tracheotome
Salyer modification of Obwegeser's mandibular procedure
Sam Roberts
   esophagoscope, S.
   headrest, S.
   self-retaining laryngoscope, S.
Samonara palatoplasty
sand

sand *(continued)*
   auditory s.
Sanchez-Bulnes lacrimal sac retractor
Sanders
   intubation laryngoscope, S.
   jet ventilation device respirator, S.
sandpaper
   dermabrader, s.
   disk, s.
sandpapering
Sandstrom glands
sandwich biopsy
Sandwith bald tongue
Sanger Brown ataxia
sanguineous
Santorini
   cartilage, S.
   fissure, S.
   incisura, S.
   ligament, S.
Sanvenero-Rosselli repair
Sappey
   fibers, S.
   ligament, S.
sarcoid
sarcoidosis
sarcoma
sardonic
   laugh, s.
SAS (sleep apnea syndrome)
SASMAS (skin-adipose superficial musculoaponeurotic system)
   face-lift, S.
Satchmo syndrome
Satellight microsurgical instruments
satellite abscess
satyr ear
saucerization
saucerize
Sauer
   speculum, S.
   tonsillectome, S.
Sauer-Sluder tonsillectome
Sauer-Wiener intranasal speculum
Saunders sign
Saunders-Paparella

Saunders-Paparella *(continued)*
   pick, S.
   stapes hook, S.
   window rasp, S.
Savary esophageal dilator
Savary-Gilliard esophageal dilator
Savin technique
saw
   bayonet s.
   separating s.
Sawtell
   nasal applicator, S.
   tonsillar forceps, S.
Sawtell-Davis tonsillar hemostat forceps
Sayoc technique
scabbard trachea
scala
   Lowenberg, s. of
   media, s.
   tympani, s.
   vestibuli, s.
scaler
   chisel s.
   deep s.
   double-ended s.
   hoe s.
   sickle s.
   superficial s.
   ultrasonic s.
scaling
   deep s.
   root s.
   subgingival s.
   ultrasonic s.
scalprum
scamping speech
scanning speech
scapha (pl. scaphae)
scaphae (pl. of scapha)
scaphoconchal
   angle, s.
scaphoid
   facies, s.
   fossa, s.
scar revision
scarlatina

scarlet fever
Scarpa
   fluid, S.
   foramen, S.
   ganglion, S.
   hiatus, S.
   membrane, S.
   nerve, S.
SCCHN (squamous cell carcinoma of head and neck)
Schaeffer
   ethmoid curette, S.
   mastoid curette, S.
Schaffer curette
Schall tube
Schantz sinus raspatory
Schatzki esophageal ring
Schatzmann attachment
Scheibe deafness
Scheie syndrome
Scheinmann laryngeal forceps
scheroma
Schilder disease
Schimek technique
Schindler esophagoscope
schindylesis
Schirmer test
schistasis
schistocephalus
schistoglossia
schistoprosopia
schistotrachelus
schizencephaly
schizoprosopia
Schlesinger solution
Schmeden
   nasal punch, s.
   tonsillar punch, S.
Schmiedel ganglion
Schmincke tumor
Schmithhuisen
   ethmoid punch, S.
   sphenoid punch, S.
Schmutz pyorrhea
schneiderian membrane
Schnidt

Schnidt *(continued)*
   hemostat, S.
   tonsillar forceps, S.
Schonbein operation
Schosser treatment
Schoemaker
   goiter scissors, S.
   line, S.
Schovinger-type incision
Schreger
   lines, S.
   striae, S.
Schuchardt-Pfeiffer procedure
Schuknecht
   excavator, S.
   footplate hook, s.
   gouge, S.
   knife, S.
   operation, S.
   piston prosthesis, S.
   retractor, S.
   speculum, S.
   stapes excavator, S.
   stapedectomy, S.
   Teflon crimper, S.
   Teflon wire piston prosthesis, S.
   trephine, S.
   wire crimper, S.
   wire-fat stapedectomy, S.
Schulex chin-plasty
Schuller
   position, S.
   view, S.
Schult disease
Schultze
   cells, S.
   sign, S.
Schultze-Chvostek sign
Schwabach test
Schwalbe corpuscle
schwannoma
Schwartze
   procedure, S.
   sign, S.
Schwarz
   activator, S.

Schwarz *(continued)*
   appliance, S.
scintigraphic
scintigraphy
scissors-bite
   crossbite, s.
sclerosant
sclerosed
sclerosing
   mastoiditis, s.
   sinusitis, s.
   solution, s.
sclerosis
sclerotherapy
sclerotic
   dentin, s.
   mastoiditis, s.
   teeth, s.
scoop
   ear s.
   mastoid s.
SCOOP 1 and 2 transtracheal catheters
scorbutic gingivitis
Scott
   attachment, S.
   cannula, S.
   speculum, S.
screw elevator
screwdriver teeth
scribing studs
scrim (speech discrimination)
scrofulous rhinitis
scroll ear
scrotal tongue
scurvy
scute
   tympanic s.
scutiform cartilage
SD (septal defect)
seal
   border s.
   double s.
   posterior palatal s.
   velopharyngeal s.
sealant
   dental s.

sealant *(continued)*
    fissure s.
    pit and fissure s.
sealer
    endodontic s.
    root canal s.
searcher
    mastoid s.
Searcy tonsillectome
seasickness
seasonal allergy
seat
    basal s.
    rest s.
seating of denture
sebaceous adenoma
Sebileau hollow
Sechrist IV-100 infant ventilator
secodont
second pharyngeal pouch
secondary
    bronchitis, s.
    dentin, s.
    dentition, s.
    teeth, s.
secretory otitis media (SOM)
Sedillot operation
SEE (Seeing Essential English)
Seeing Essential English (SEE)
see-saw nystagmus
Seessel
    pocket, S.
    pouch, S.
Segura procedure for esophageal varices
Seiffert forceps
Seiler
    formula, S.
    tonsillar knife, S.
    turbinate scissors, S.
Seitz metamorphosing respiration
Seldane
selenodont
self
    -curing resin, s.
    -medicate, s.
    -medication, s.

sella
    turcica, s.
sellar
Sellick maneuver
semantic aphasia
semicanal
    auditory tube, s. of
    tensor tympani muscle, s. of
semicanales
semicanalis
    musculi tensoris tympani, s.
    tubae auditivae, s.
semicircular
    canal, s.
    duct, s.
semicrista
    incisiva, s.
semilunar
    canal, s.
    incision, s.
Semken forceps
Semon
    law, S.
    sign, S.
Semon-Rosenbach law
Sengstaken
    balloon, S.
    tube, S.
Sengstaken-Blakemore tube
Senn mastoid retractor
Senn-Dingman retractor
sensitization
sensitized
sensorimotor
sensorineural
    deafness, s.
    hearing loss. s. (SSNHL)
sensory
    amusia, s.
    aphasia, s.
sentinel node
Senturia speculum
SEO (severe external otitis)
separator
septa (pl. of septum)
septal

septal *(continued)*
  annuloplasty, s.
  cartilage, s.
  chisel, s.
  defect, s. (SD)
  deflection, s.
  deviation, s.
  elevator, s.
  fracture, s.
  gingiva, s.
  gouge, s.
  knife, s.
  punch, s.
  ridge, s.
  splint, s.
  straightener, s.
  trephine, s.
septate
septation
septectomy
septic
  sore throat, s.
septile
Septisol
septomarginal
septometer
septometry
septonasal
septoplasty
septostomy
septotome
septotomy
septum (pl. septa)
  auditory tube, s. of
  bony s. of eustachian canal
  bony s. of nose
  bronchial s.
  enamel s.
  frontal sinuses, s. of
  gingival s.
  gum s.
  interalveolar s.
  interdental s.
  lingual s.
  membranous s. of nose
  nasal s.

septum (pl. septa) *(continued)*
  nasi osseum, s.
  orbital s.
  pharyngeal s.
  sphenoidal sinuses, s. of
  tongue, s. of
  tracheoesophageal s.
  tubae, s.
septum chisel
septum clamp
septum elevator
septum forceps
septum knife
septum straightener
septum-straightening forceps
sequestration
sequestrectomy
sequestrotomy
seriflux
seromembranous
seromucoid
seromucous
  gland, s.
seromucus
seropurulent
seropus
serosanguineous
serous
  drainage, s.
  effusion, s.
  exudate, s.
  inflammation, s.
  membrane, s.
  otitis media, s. (SOM)
serrated
serration
Serres
  angle, S.
  glands, S.
  operation, S.
serumal calculus
sesamoid
  cartilage, s.
setback
setup
  diagnostic s.

setup wax
severe external otitis (SEO)
Sewall
    antral cannula, S.
    antral trocar, S.
    ethmoidal chisel, S.
    mucoperiosteal elevator, S.
    raspatory, S.
Sewell-Boyden flap
sextant
Sexton bayonet ear knife
sexual asthma
SGV (salivary gland virus)
shadow curve
shadow-free laryngoscope
Shallcross
    nasal-packing forceps, S.
    tonsillar hemostat, S.
shallow
    breathing, s.
    respirations, s.
sham-movement vertigo
Shambaugh
    adenotome, S.
    endaural elevator, S.
    fistula hook, S.
    headrest, S.
    hook, S.
    incision, S.
    irrigator, S.
    needle, S.
    retractor, S.
    technique, S.
Shambaugh-Derlacki
    chisel, S.
    endaural elevator, S.
Shambaugh-Lempert knife
shank
Shapleigh ear curette
Shapshay/Healy 20 cm phonatory and operating laryngoscope
Sharpey perforating fibers
Shaw scalpel
Shea
    bail-hook prosthesis, S.
    curette, S.

Shea *(continued)*
    ear drill, S.
    footplate hook, s.
    irrigator, S.
    knife, S.
    malleus gripper prosthesis, S.
    stapedectomy, S.
    Teflon piston prosthesis, S.
    tube, S.
    vein-polyethylene strut stapedectomy, S.
Shea-Anthony antral balloon
Shearer forceps
sheath
    carotid s.
    dentinal s.
    Neumann, s. of
shedding
Sheehan nasal chisel
Sheehy
    button, S.
    canal knife, S.
    collar-button tube, S.
    incus replacement prosthesis, S.
    ossicle-holding clamp, S.
    syndrome, S.
    tube, S.
Sheehy-House incus replacement prosthesis
Sheen rhinoplasty
Sheinmann laryngeal forceps
shelf
    buccal s.
    dental s.
    palatine s.
shell
    crown, s.
    tooth, s.
shellac bases
Shepard
    collar-button tube, S.
    grommet tube, S.
Sherman plate
Shiley
    endotracheal tube, S.
    tracheostomy tube, S.

shirt-stud abscess
short increment sensitivity index (SISI)
short process
    incus, s. of
    malleus, s. of
shotty nodes
shovel-shaped incisors
Shrapnell membrane
Shrapshay/Healey 20 cm. phonatory and operating laryngoscope
siagantritis
siagonagra
siagonantritis
sialaden
sialadenitis
    chronic nonspecific s.
sialadenography
sialadenoncus
sialadenosis
sialadenotomy
sialagogic
sialagogue
sialaporia
sialectasia
sialectasis
sialemesis
sialic
sialine
sialism
sialismus
sialitis
sialoadenectomy
sialoadenolithotomy
sialoadenotomy
sialoaerophagia
sialoaerophagy
sialoangiectasis
sialoangiitis
sialoangiography
sialocele
sialodochiectas
sialodochitis
    fibrinosa, s.
sialodochoplasty
sialoductitis
sialogastrone

sialogenous
sialogogic
sialogogue
sialogram
sialography
sialolith
sialolithiasis
sialolithotomy
sialoma
sialometaplasia
    necrotizing s.
sialomucin
sialoncus
sialophagia
sialoporia
sialorrhea
sialoschesis
sialosemeiology
sialosis
sialotic
sialostenosis
sialosyrinx
sialozemia
sibilant
    breath sounds, s.
    rales, s.
sibilance
sibilation
sibilismus
    aurium, s.
sibilus
Sibileau hollow
sickle
    middle-ear knife, s.
    scaler, s.
    tonsillar knife, s.
side
    balancing s.
    functioning s.
    nonfunctioning s.
    working s.
side mouth gag
sideropenic dysphagia
Siegel otoscope
Siegle otoscope
Sierra-Sheldon tracheotome

sigh
sighing
   respirations, s.
sigma angle
sigmoid sinus
sign language
signed
signing
Siker laryngoscope
Silastic
   glenoid fossa prosthesis, S.
   grommet, S.
   keel of vomer, S.
   patch, S.
   sheeting, S.
   thyroid drain, S.
silent
   mastoiditis, s.
   thyroiditis, s.
silex
silica
silicate cement
silicophosphate cement
Silvadene
silver
   chisel, s.
   crown, s.
   filling, s.
   nitrate, s.
   nitrate cautery, s.
   point method, s.
   points, s.
   wire, s.
Silver
   osteotome, S.
   skin graft knife, S.
   syndrome, S.
Silver-Hildreth eyelid operation
Simon cheiloplasty
simple
   anchorage, s.
   mastoidectomy, s.
   sinusotomy, s.
Simplex mastoid rongeur
Simpson antral curette
SIN (squamous intraepithelial neoplasia)

sinal
sinapism
Singapore ear
Singer-Blom
   electrolarynx prosthesis, S.
   valve, S.
singer's
   node, s.
   nodule, s.
single
   -bevel chisel, s.
   cone method, s.
singultation
singultous
singultus
sinistrality
sinistraural
sinobronchitis
sinodural
sinogram
sinography
sinonasal
sinopulmonary
Sinskey hook
sinuitis
sinuotomy
sinus
   accessory nasal s's
   branchial s.
   Breschet s.
   carotid s.
   cavernosus, s.
   cavernous s.
   cochleae, s.
   draining s.
   ethmoidal s's
   ethmoidalis, s.
   frontal s.
   frontalis osseus, s.
   Huguier s.
   intercavernous s.
   laryngeal s.
   lymph s's
   Maier, s. of
   mastoid s.
   maxillaris highmori, s.

sinus *(continued)*
    maxillaris osseus, s.
    maxillary s.
    medii, s.
    Meyeri, s.
    Meyer s.
    Morgani, s. of
    occipital s.
    oral s.
    paranasal s's
    paranasales, s.
    petrosal s.
    piriform s.
    posterior cavi tympani, s.
    Ridley s.
    sigmoid s.
    sphenoidal s's
    sphenoidalis, s.
    sphenoidalis osseus, s.
    sphenoparietal s.
    tonsillar s.
    tympani, s.
    tympanic s.
sinus balloon
sinus barotrauma
sinus block
sinus bur
sinus cannula
sinus catarrh
sinus chisel
sinus clouding
sinus curette
sinus drainage
sinus films
sinus floor
sinus groove
sinus infection
sinus-irrigating cannula
sinus ostia
sinus probe
sinus rasp
sinus series
sinus tract
sinus tympani
sinus tympanicus
sinus wash bottle
sinusal
sinusitis
    acute catarrhal s.
    acute suppurative s.
    chronic hypertrophic s.
    ethmoid s.
    frontal s.
    fungal s.
    hyperplastic s.
    intracranial s.
    maxillary s.
    orbital s.
    sphenoid s.
    viral s.
sinusoid
    lymph node, s.
sinusoidal
sinusoidalization
sinusotomy
Sippy esophageal dilator
Sirognathograph Analysing System
SISI (short increment sensitivity index)
Sisson-Cottle septal speculum
Sisson-Vienna nasal speculum
Sistrunk operation
situs
    inversus, s.
sixth-year molar
Sjogren syndrome
skeletal analysis
skew deviation
Skillern
    sinus probe, S.
    sphenoid probe, S.
skin pencil
Skin Skribe
skin
    adipose superficial
        musculoaponeurotic system, s.
        (SASMAS)
    crease, s.
    flap, s.
    fold, s.
    graft, s.
    hook, s.
    paddle, s.

skin *(continued)*
   pencil, s.
   planing, s.
   pocket, s.
   sleeve, s.
skinfold
   caliper, s.
   incision, s.
Skinner classification
Skoog
   cleft lip repair, S.
   nasal chisel, S.
skull
   base, s.
   plate, s.
Slaughter nasal saw
sleep apnea
   syndrome, s. (SAS)
sleeve procedure
sliding
   flap, s.
   genoplasty, s.
   hiatal hernia, s.
   laryngoscope, s.
sling
   attachment, s.
slope
   lower ridge s.
   mandibular anteroposterior ridge s.
slot dome incision
slotted
   bronchoscope, s.
   laryngoscope, s.
slough
sloughing
   skin, s. of
Sluder
   adenotome, S.
   hook, S.
   method, S.
   mouth gag, S.
   neuralgia, S.
   palate retractor, S.
   speculum, S.
   tonsillar guillotine, S.
   tonsillectome, S.

Sluder *(continued)*
   tonsillectomy, S.
Sluder-Ballenger tonsillectome
Sluder-Demarest tonsillectome
Sluder-Ferguson mouth gag
Sluder-Jansen mouth gag
Sluder-Sauer
   tonsillar guillotine, S.
   tonsillectome, S.
slurred speech
small airways
   dysfunction, s.
smas layer
SMAS (superficial musculoaponeurotic system)
   face-lift technique, S.
   level, S.
smell-brain
Smith tonsillar dissector
Smith-Lemli-Opitz syndrome
Smithuysen
   ethmoidal punch, S.
   sphenoidal punch, S.
smoke inhalation
smoker's
   bronchitis, s.
   cancer, s.
   cough, s.
   palate, s.
   patches, s.
   pharynx, s.
   tongue, s.
smoking
   history, s.
   passive s.
SMR (submucous resection)
   speculum, S.
SMRR (submucous resection and rhinoplasty)
SNA (sella, nasion, reference point A)
snaggle tooth
snare
   cautery, s.
   technique, s.
   tonsillectomy, s.
   wire, s.

SNB (sella, nasion, reference point B)
sneeze
   reflex, s.
sneezing
Snellen
   reflex, S.
   technique, S.
   test, S.
SSNHL (sudden sensorineural hearing loss)
sniffles
sniffling
   bronchophony, s.
Snitman endaural retractor
snore
snoring
snuff
snuffles
snuffling
snugged up
SOAE (spontaneous otoacoustic emission)
sob
socia parotidis
socioacusis
socket
   alveolar s.
   dry s.
   tooth s.
Soemmering
   bone, S.
   process, S.
soft
   cervical collar, s.
   chancre, s.
   collar, s.
   diet, s.
   palate, s.
   palate retractor, s.
solar cheilitis
solder
   building s.
   gold s.
   hard s.
   soft s.
soldered

soldering
solid-state esophageal manometry catheter
Solis-Cohen laryngectomy
solitary bone cyst
solum tympani
solution
   lactated Ringer's s.
   normal saline s.
   physiological saline s.
   Ringer's s.
   saline s.
   sclerosing s.
Solvang graft
SOM (secretory otitis media or serous otitis media)
SOMI (sternal-occipital-mandibular immobilization) brace
sone
sonic boom
sonicate
sonitus
Sonneberg operation
Sonnenschein nasal speculum
sonometer
Sophy programmable pressure valve
sordes
sore
   canker s.
   cold s.
sore throat
   clergyman's s.
   diphtheritic s.
   epidemic streptococcal s.
   Fothergill s.
   hospital s.
   putrid s.
   quinsy s.
   septic s.
   spotted s.
   streptococcal s.
   ulcerated s.
Sorenson sinus cleanser
sound
   pressure level, s. (SPL)
Sourdille operation
Souttar tube

space
- Cotunnius s.
- dentin, s's in
- epitympanic s.
- escapement s's
- Henke s.
- interarytenoid s.
- interdental s.
- interocclusal s.
- interproximal s.
- interproximate s.
- interradicular s.
- Kiesselbach s.
- Kretschmann s.
- lymph s.
- Nance leeway s.
- parapharyngeal s.
- peripharyngeal s.
- pharyngomaxillary s.
- proximal s.
- proximate s.
- Prussak s.
- relief s.
- retromyelohyoid s.
- retropharyngeal s.
- septal s.
- subgingival s.
- submaxillary s.
- thyrohyal s.
- Troltsch s.

space maintainer
spacer
Spaeth technique
spasm
- Bell s.
- bronchial s.
- bronchopulmonary s.
- canine s.
- coughing s.
- cynic s.
- diffuse esophageal s.
- esophageal s.
- facial s.
- glottic s.
- habit s.
- histrionic s.

spasm *(continued)*
- inspiratory s.
- laryngeal s.
- nictitating s.
- nodding s.
- paroxysmal coughing s.
- phonatory s.
- respiratory s.
- rotatory s.
- salaam s.
- winking s.

spasmatic
- asthma, s.
- croup, s.
- stricture, s.

spasmodic
- asthma, s.
- cough, s.
- croup, s.
- torticollis, s.

spasmogen
spasmology
spasmolygmus
spasmolysin
spasmolytic
spasmophemia
spasmous
spasmus
- bronchialis, s.
- caninus, s.
- coordinatus, s.
- cynicus, s.
- Dubini, s.
- glottidis, s.
- nictitans, s.
- nutans, s.

spastic
- aphonia, s.

spasticity
spatula
- dental s.
- mallei, s.
- nasal s.

spatulate
speaking tube
spec (speculum)

spec (speculum) *(continued)*
    exam, s.
special sense organs
speckled
    erythroplasia, s.
    leukoplakia, s.
Spectra-Physics argon laser
speculum
    ear s.
speech
    alaryngeal s.
    aphonic s.
    ataxic s.
    audiometry, s.
    clipped s.
    echo s.
    esophageal s.
    explosive s.
    incoherent s.
    interjectional s.
    jumbled s.
    mirror s.
    plateau s.
    pressured s.
    scamping s.
    scanning s.
    slurring s.
    staccato s.
speech abnormality
speech-aid prosthesis
speech bulb
speech discrimination
speech disorder
speech impediment
speech pathologist
speech-reading
speech reception test (SRT)
speech reception threshold (SRT)
speech synthesizer
speech therapist
speech therapy
sphagiasmus
sphagitides
sphagitis
Spencer
    labyrinth probe, S.

Spencer *(continued)*
    punch, S.
sphenethmoid
sphenion
sphenobasilar
sphenoccipital
sphenocephalus
sphenoethmoid
sphenoethmoidal
    recess, s.
    suture, s.
sphenoethmoidectomy
sphenofrontal
    suture, s.
sphenoid
    air sinuses, s.
    body, s.
    bone, s.
    sinusotomy, s.
sphenoidal
    angle, s.
    bur, s.
    concha, s.
    crest, s.
    fissure, s.
    fontanelle, s.
    joint, s.
    knife, s.
    paranasal sinus, s.
    probe, s.
    ridge, s.
    rostrum, s.
    spine, s.
    structures, s.
    strut, s.
    turbinate, s.
    turbinated processes, s.
    wing, s.
    yoke, s.
sphenoidectomy
    frontoethmoid s.
sphenoiditis
sphenoidostomy
sphenoidotomy
sphenomalar
    suture, s.

sphenomandibular
sphenomaxillary
  fissure, s.
  fossa, s.
  ganglion, s.
  suture, s.
spheno-occipital
spheno-orbital
sphenopalatine
  canal, s.
  foramen, s.
  ganglion, s.
  ganglionectomy, s.
  needle, s.
  notch, s.
sphenoparietal
  sinus, s.
  suture, s.
sphenopetrosal
sphenopharyngeal
  canal, s.
sphenopterygoid
  canal, s.
sphenorbital
sphenosalpingostaphylinus
sphenosquamosal
sphenosquamous
sphenotemporal
  suture, s.
sphenotic
sphenoturbinal
sphenovomerine
sphenozygomatic
  suture, s.
spheresthesia
sphincter
  esophageal s.
  incompetent esophageal s.
  oris, s.
  palatopharyngeal s.
  pharyngoesophageal s.
Spiegler-Fendt sarcoid
Spielberg sinus cannula
Spies ethmoidal punch
Spina cleft lip repair
spinal

spinal *(continued)*
  accessory nerve, s.
  fluid, s.
  fluid rhinorrhea, s.
spine
  anterior maxillary s.
  basilar s.
  ethmoidal s.
  ethmoidal s. of Macalister
  frontal bone s.
  Henle, s. of
  maxillary s.
  meatal s.
  mental s.
  nasal s.
  palatine s's
  pharyngeal s.
  sphenoidal s.
  suprameatal s.
  trochlear s.
  tympanic s.
spinning sensation
spiral
  canal of cochlea, s.
  canal of modiolus, s.
  crest of cochlea, s.
  lamina, s.
  organ of Corti, s.
spiroid canal
spirometer
spirometry
  incentive s.
spissated
spissitude
spit
spittle
SPL (sound pressure level)
splayed
splaying
spline
  stapes s.
splint
  acrylic resin bite-guard s.
  anchor s.
  dental s.
  permanent fixed s.

splint *(continued)*
   temporary removable s.
split
   cast method, s.
   osteotomy, s.
   plate appliance, s.
   -rib bone graft, s.
   tongue, s.
spoken voice test
spondee
Spondel foramen
spondylosis
spondylotic
spongy gums
spontaneous otoacoustic emission (SOAE)
spoon
   excavator, s.
Spratt
   ear curette, S.
   mastoid curette, S.
   raspatory, S.
spreader
   root canal s.
sprue
spud
spur
   malleus, s. of
spurious torticollis
spurred
spurring
sputa (pl. of sputum)
sputamentum
sputum (pl. sputa)
   aeroginosum, s.
   albuminoid s.
   blood-tinged s.
   bloody s.
   coctum, s.
   crudum, s.
   cruentum, s.
   frothy s.
   globular s.
   green s.
   icteric s.
   moss-agate s.

sputum (pl. sputa) *(continued)*
   mucopurulent s.
   nummular s.
   productive s.
   prune-juice s.
   purulent s.
   rusty s.
   septicemia s.
   tenacious s.
sputum collection
sputum cytology
sputum production
sputum smear
sputum specimen
sputum tube
squama (pl. squamae)
squamae (pl. of squama)
squame
squamocolumnar junction, s.
squamofrontal
squamomastoid
squamo-occipital
squamoparietal
squamopetrosal
squamosa
squamosal
squamosomastoid
squamosoparietal
squamosphenoid
squamotemporal
squamous
   cell, s.
   cell carcinoma of head and neck, s. (SCCHN)
   epithelium, s.
   intraepithelial neoplasia, s. (SIN)
   suture, s.
squamozygomatic
squint angle
SRT (speech reception test OR threshold)
stabilization
staccato
   cough, s.
   speech, s.
Stacke mastoidectomy

Stader splint
Stafne defect
staggering
Stahl ear
Stahr gland
Stailine Super-EBA cement
stainless steel
    bobbin, s.
    piston, s.
    plate, s.
    prosthesis, s.
    strut, s.
    wire, s.
Stallard conjunctivocystorhinostomy
Stammberger antrum punch
stannous fluoride
stapedectomy
    forceps, s.
    knife, s.
stapedial
    ankylosis, s.
    crus, s.
    fold, s.
    footplate auger, s.
    nerve, s.
    tendon, s.
stapediolysis
stapedioplasty
stapediotenotomy
stapediovestibular
stapedius
    muscle, s.
    nerve, s.
    tendon, s.
stapes
    annular ligament of s.
    chisel, s.
    curette, s.
    dilator, s.
    elevator, s.
    excavator, s.
    fixation of s.
    footplate, s.
    hoe, s.
    hook, s.
    measuring device, s.

stapes *(continued)*
    mobilization, s.
    pick, s.
    piston, s.
    prosthesis, s.
    speculum, s.
    spline, s.
    superstructure, s.
    tapping hammer, s.
    wire guide, s.
staph (staphylococcus)
    bronchitis, s.
    infection, s.
staphylagra
staphyle
staphylectomy
staphyledema
staphylematoma
staphyline glands
staphylinus
staphylion
staphylitis
staphyloangina
staphylococcal
Staphylococcus
    aureus, S.
staphylodialysis
staphyloncus
staphylopharyngorrhaphy
staphyloplasty
staphyloptosia
staphyloptosis
staphylorrhaphy
    elevator, s.
    needle, s.
staphyloschisis
staphylotome
staphylotomy
staphylotoxin
Stark technique
starry-sky pattern
static equilibrium
stationary
    anchorage, s.
    bridge, s.
    lingual arch, s.

statoacoustic
statoconia (pl. of statoconium)
statoconium (pl. statoconia)
statocyst
statokinetic labyrinth
statolith
status
   asthmaticus, s.
   epilepticus, s.
   parathyreoprivus, s.
   sternuens, s.
   vertiginosus, s.
staurion
St. Clair-Thompson
   adenotome, S.
   curette, S.
   peritonsillar abscess forceps, S.
steam
   fitters' asthma, s.
   inhalation, s.
   tent, s.
Steele bronchial dilator
Steffanoff ear reconstruction
Stein
   cheiloplasty, S.
   operation, S.
   test, S.
Stein-Abbe lip flap
Steiner plane
Steinhauser Titanium bone plate system
Steinmann pin
Stenger test
stenion
Steno
   canal, S.
   duct, S.
stenosis
   esophageal s.
   laryngeal s.
   subglottic s.
   tracheal s.
stenotic
Stensen
   canal, S.
   duct, S.
   foramen, S.

Stensen *(continued)*
   plexus, S.
stent
   dressing, s.
   graft, s.
stented
stenting
Stenver
   position, S.
   view, S.
step-off of facial bones
stephanion
stepped cylinder
sterculia gum
Steri-Strip
steri-stripped
sternoclavicular
sternocleidomastoid
sternocleidomastoideus
sternohyoid
   bursa, s.
steroid
   facies, s.
sternomastoid
sternothyroid
sternotracheal
Sterns attachment
sternutatio
   convulsiva, s.
sternutation
   convulsive s.
sternutator
sternutatory
stertor
stertorous
   respiration, s.
Stevens scissors
Stevens-Johnson syndrome
Stevenson-LaForce adenotome
stiff neck
stillicidium
   lacrimarium, s.
   narium, s.
Stillman cleft
stimulant expectorant
Stinger test

stippled tongue
stirrup
  bone, s.
stithe
Stoerk blennorrhea
Stoker treatment
Stokes expectorant
stoma (pl. stomata)
  tracheostomy, s.
stomacace
stomach
  cough, s.
  tooth, s.
stomachal vertigo
stomata (pl. of stoma)
stomatalgia
stomatic
stomatitides (pl. of stomatitis)
stomatitis (pl. stomatitides)
  allergic s.
  angular s.
  aphthous s.
  arsenicalis, s.
  bismuth s.
  catarrhal s.
  contact s.
  corrosive s.
  denture s.
  diphtheritic s.
  epidemic s.
  erythematopultaceous s.
  exanthematica, s.
  follicular s.
  fusospirochetal s.
  gangrenous s.
  gonococcal s.
  gonorrheal s.
  herpetic s.
  infectious s.
  intertropica, s.
  lead s.
  medicamentosa, s.
  membranous s.
  mercurial s.
  mycotic s.
  nicotina, s.

stomatitis (pl. stomatitides) *(continued)*
  nonspecific s.
  parasitica, s.
  recurrent aphthous s.
  scarlatina, s.
  scorbutica, s.
  simple s.
  syphilitic s.
  traumatic s.
  tropical s.
  ulcerative s.
  uremic s.
  venenata, s.
  vesicular s.
  Vincent s.
stomatocace
stomatodynia
stomatodysodia
stomatoglossitis
stomatognathic
stomatography
stomatolalia
stomatologist
stomatology
stomatomalacia
stomatomenia
stomatomycosis
stomatonecrosis
stomatonoma
stomatopathy
stomatoplasty
stomatorrhagia
  gingivarum, s.
stomatoschisis
stomatoscope
stomion
stomocephalus
stomodeal
stomodeum
stomoschisis
stone
  dental s.
  red s.
  salivary s.
stone asthma
stop-valve airway obstruction

Storm Van Leeuwen chamber
Storz
   anterior commissure laryngoscope, S.
   bronchoscope, S.
   esophageal conductor, S.
   folding emergency ventilation bronchoscope, S.
   folding-handle ear knife, S.
   infant bronchoscope, S.
   intratracheal tube, S.
   laryngopharyngoscope, S.
   nasal speculum, S.
   nasopharyngeal biopsy forceps, S.
   optical esophagoscope, S.
   sinus biopsy forceps, S.
Storz-Beck tenaculum
Storz-Bruenings ear magnifier
Storz-Doesel-Huzly bronchoscope tube
Storz-Hopkins laryngoscope
Storz-LaForce adenotome
Storz-LaForce-Stevenson adenotome
Stout wiring
straddling dermabrasion
straight-blade laryngoscope
Straith
   otoplasty, S.
   profilometer, S.
strangle
strangulated
strangulation
strap muscles
strawberry tongue
strep (streptococcus)
   EIA, s.
   ID, s.
   screen, s.
   throat, s.
   URI, s.
streptococcal
   bronchitis, s.
   tonsillitis, s.
Streptococcus
   viridans, S.
stress-bearing area
stria (pl. striae)
   vascularis ductus cochlearis, s.

striae (pl. of stria)
stricture
strictured
strident
stridor
   dentium, s.
   laryngeal s.
   respiratory s.
   serraticus, s.
stridulous
Stringer newborn throat forceps
stripe
   paratracheal s.
stripper's asthma
stripping of vocal cords
Stroud excision of external ear
structure
   denture-supporting s.
Struempel ear alligator forceps
Struempel-Voss ethmoidal forceps
struma
   aberranta, s.
   cast iron s.
   colloides, s.
   congenita, s.
   Hashimoto s.
   lingualis, s.
   lymphomatosa, s.
   maligna, s.
   nodosa, s.
   Riedel s.
strumectomy
strumiprivous
strumitis
strumous
strut
   bar, s.
   calibration, s.
   calipers, s.
   graft, s.
   hook, s.
   pick, s.
   rhinoplasty, s.
Struyken
   nasal cutting forceps, S.
   turbinate forceps, S.

Stryker
   dermatome, S.
   saw, S.
Stubbs adenoid curette
stud
study cast
stuffy nose
Stutsman snare
stutter
stuttering
stylette
styletted tracheobronchial catheter
styloglossus
stylohyal
stylohyoid
stylohyoideus
styloid
   process, s.
styloiditis
stylomandibular
   ligament, s.
stylomastoid
   foramen, s.
stylomaxillary
stylomyloid
stylopharyngeus
stylostaphyline
stylosteophyte
stylus tracing
stype
styptic
   cotton, s.
   pencil, s.
styrene resin
St. Vitus dance of the voice
subapical
   osteotomy, s.
subarachnoid
subaural
subaurale
subauricular
subciliary
subclavian
subcondylar
   osteotomy, s.
subcortical aphasia

subdental
subdural abscess
subepiglottic
subgemmal
subgingival
   calculus, s.
   curettage, s.
subglossal
subglossitis
subglottic
   chink, s.
   hemangioma, s.
   laryngitis, s.
   stenosis, s.
subhyoid
   bursa, s.
   pharyngotomy, s.
subhyoidean
subiculum
subjacent
sublabial
   adhesion, s.
sublingual
   caruncle, s.
   crescent, s.
   duct, s.
   fold, s.
   gland, s.
   saliva, s.
   tablet, s.
sublinguitis
submandibular
   duct, s.
   gland, s.
   lymph nodes, s.
   salivary gland, s.
submandibularitis
submantle layer
submaxilla
submaxillaritis
submaxillary
   duct of Wharton, s.
   ganglion, s.
   gland, s.
   space, s.
   triangle, s.

submental
  gland, s.
  lymph node, s.
submerged
  tonsil, s.
  tooth, s.
submucosa
submucosal
submucous
  curette, s.
  dissection, s.
  dissector, s.
  elevator, s.
  knife, s.
  resection, s. (SMR)
  resection and rhinoplasty, s. (SMRR)
  retractor, s.
submucous resection (SMR)
subnasal
subnasale
subnasion
suboccipital
subocclusal
subodontoblastic
  layer, s.
suborbital
subparietal
subperiosteal
  abscess, s.
  implant, s.
subpharyngeal
subpulpal
subpyramidal
subsibilant
subspinale
substantia (pl. substantiae)
  adamantina dentis, s.
  eburnea dentis, s.
substantiae (pl. of substantia)
substernomastoid
substructure
  implant s.
subtrochlear
subtympanic
subvomerine cartilage
subzygomatic

succedaneous teeth
successional teeth
succorrhea
suck
sucking pad
suction
  nasogastric s.
  nasotracheal s.
suctioning
suctorial pad
suffocant
suffocate
suffocation
suffocative
  bronchitis, s.
  catarrh, s.
  goiter, s.
Sugiura
  devascularization of esophagus and stomach, S.
  esophageal varices, S.
  procedure, S.
sulcated tongue
sulci (pl. of sulcus)
sulcular epithelium
sulcus (pl. sulci)
  alveololingual s.
  antihelicis transversus, s.
  ethmoid s. of Gegenbaur
  eustachian tube, s. of
  gingival s.
  greater palatine s.
  infraorbital s.
  Jacobson s.
  labiodental s.
  lacrimal s.
  mallear s.
  mandibular s.
  mastoid caniculus, s. of
  mentolabial s.
  mylohyoid s. of mandible
  nasal s.
  nasolabial s.
  olfactory s.
  palatine s. of maxilla
  palatovaginal s.

sulcus (pl. sulci) *(continued)*
   petrobasilar s.
   petrosal s.
   pterygoid s.
   pterygopalatine s.
   sigmoid s.
   sinus transversi, s.
   spiralis, s.
   supraorbital s.
   tongue, s. of
   tubae auditoriae, s.
   tympanic s.
   vomeral s.
   vomerovaginal s.
sulfanilamide crystals
Sulfamylon
Sullivan
   raspatory, S.
   sinus rasp, S.
Summerskill dacryocystorhinostomy
summit of nose
Sunday staphylorrhaphy elevator
sunset eyes
superaurale
superficial
   musculoaponeurotic system, s. (SMAS)
   temporal artery, s.
Superglue
superior
   carotid triangle, s.
   dental nerve, s.
   lingualis muscle, s.
   maxillary nerve, s.
   nasal concha, s.
   nuchal line, s.
   petrosal sinus, s.
   semicircular canal, s.
   tympanic artery, s.
   vocal cords, s.
supermaxilla
supernumerary teeth
supersphenoid
superstructure
   implant s.
supporting cells

suppressant
suppression
suppuration
suppurative
   marginal gingivitis, s.
   mastoiditis, s.
   otochondritis, s.
   tonsillitis, s.
supra-arytenoid cartilage
supra-auricular
suprabuccal
suprabulge
supraciliary canal
supraclavicular
supraclusion
supracondylar
supragingival
   calculus, s.
supraglottic
   larynx, s.
supraglottitis
suprahyoid
supramandibular
supramastoid
   crest, s.
supramaxilla
supramaxillary
suprameatal
   spine, s.
   triangle, s.
supramental
supramentale
supranasal
supranuclear paralysis
supraocclusion
supraomohyoid neck dissection
supraoptic canal
supraorbital
   arch, s.
   canal, s.
   neuralgia, s.
   notch, s.
supraperiosteal
suprasellar
suprastapedial
suprasternal

supratip
supratonsillar
   fossa, s.
supratympanic
supraversion
Suprax
surdimute
surdimutism
surdimutitas
surditas
   congenita, c.
surdity
surface
   alveolar s. of maxilla
   axial s.
   basal s.
   buccal s.
   contact, s's of
   distal s.
   facial s.
   foundation s.
   frontal s.
   impression s.
   incisal s.
   intratemporal s. of maxilla
   labial s.
   lateral s.
   lingual s.
   masticatory s.
   medial s.
   morsal s's
   occlusal s. of teeth
   oral s.
   polished s.
   posterior s.
   proximal s.
   proximate s.
   subocclusal s.
   superior s.
   vestibular s.
   working occlusal s.
Surgicel
survey line
suspension
   laryngoscope, s.
   laryngoscopy, s.

Sus-Phrine
suspirious
Sutton disease
sutura (pl. suturae)
suturae (pl. of sutura)
suture
   Goethe, s. of.
Suzanne gland
swab
swallow syncope
swallower
swallowing
   air s.
   painful s.
   tongue s.
swallowing center
swallowing function study
swallowing mechanism
swallowing motion
swallow's nest
swayback nose
Sweet esophageal scissors
Swenson otoplasty
swimmer's ear
swinging-door operation
swish-and-swallow mouthwash
Swiss-cheese configuration
swivel tracheostomy tube
Sydenham
   cough, S.
   mouth gag, S.
syllabic utterance
syllable stumbling
sylvian line
sympathetic saliva
sympathomimetic
symphyseal
symphyses (pl. of symphysis)
symphysis (pl. symphyses)
   jaw, s. of
   mandibular s.
   mental s.
symptomatic
   asthma, s.
   treatment, s.
synache

synchilia
synchondroses (pl. of synchondrosis)
synchondrosis (pl. synchondroses)
syncope
    carotid sinus s.
    cough s.
    laryngeal s.
    swallow s.
    tussive s.
    vasovagal s.
syncytial
syndesmo-odontoid
syndesmoses (pl. of syndesmosis)
syndesmosis (pl. syndesmoses)
synechia (pl. synechiae)
synechiae (pl. of synechia)
Syngamus
    laryngeus, S.

synotia
synotus
synovial chondromatosis
syntactical aphasia
Synthes
    facial curette, S.
    facial drill, S.
syphilitic laryngitis
syringe
    ear s.
    nasal s.
    oral s.
Syzmanowski
    otoplasty, S.
    technique, S.
    triangle method, S.

Additional entries

T

T&A (tonsillectomy and adenoidectomy)
    suction tip, T.
Tabb
    ear elevator, T.
    myringoplasty knife, T.
tabella
tabes
tabetic
    otalgia, t.
tablet
    buccal t.
    sublingual t.
tack operation of Cody
Tack sacculotomy
tactile aphasia
tag
    auricular t.
    skin t.
    tonsillar t.
tagliacotian rhinoplasty
Tagliacozzi
    flap, T.
    nasal reconstruction, T.
Taillefer valve
Takahashi
    ethmoid forceps, T.
    nasal punch, T.
talantropia
talking tracheostomy tube
tampon
    esophageal t.
    nasal t.
    tracheal t.
tamponade
    balloon t.
    esophagogastric t.
    nasal t.
tamponage
tang
Tangier disease
tank ear
Tanner mesher
Tanner-Vanderput

Tanner-Vanderput *(continued)*
    graft, T.
    mesh dermatome, T.
Tansley procedure
tantalum
    bronchogram, t.
    stapes prosthesis, t.
Tanzer auricular reconstruction
tapered crown
Tapia syndrome
tapir mouth
tapiroid
tarsectomy
tarsocheiloplasty
tarsoplasty
tarsorrhaphy
tarsus
    inferior palpebrae, t.
    superior palpebrae, t.
tartar
taste
    after-t.
    color t.
    nerves of t.
    organ of t.
taste area
taste bud
taste blindness
taste buds
taste bulb
taste cells
taste fibers
taste hairs
tasting
tattoo
tattooed
tattooing
Taub speech procedure
taurodontism
Tavist-D
Taylor Merocel ear wick
TCNS (transcutaneous nerve stimulator)
TDT (tone decay test)

TE (tracheoesophageal)
    fistula, T.
tea taster's cough
teacher's
    node, t.
    nodule, t.
Teale procedure
tear
    crocodile t's
tear duct
tear sac
tectorial
tectorium
teeth
    charting and numbering of t.
    ligation of t.
teeth ligation
teething
    lotion, t.
TEF (tracheoesophageal fistula)
Teflon
    injection, T.
    prosthesis, T.
    sheet, T.
    -wire piston, T.
tegmen (pl. tegmina)
    antri, t.
    cellulae, t.
    mastoideotympanicum, t.
    mastoideum, t.
    tympani, t.
tegmenta (pl. of tegmentum)
tegmental
tegmentum (pl. tegmenta)
    auris, t.
tegmina (pl. of tegmen)
telescope crown
telescopic denture
telescoping crossbite
Teleseal
teletactor
Teletrast
template
    occlusal t.
    wax t.
temple

tempora
temporal
    arteritis, t.
    bone, t.
    headache, t.
    line, t.
    trephine, t.
temporalis
    fascia, t.
    muscle, t.
temporary
    base, t.
    crown, t.
    filling, t.
temporoauricular
temporofacial
    graft, t.
temporofrontal
temporohyoid
temporomalar
temporomandibular (TM)
    articular clicking, t.
    articulation, t.
    fossa, t.
    joint, t. (TMJ)
    joint dysfunction, t. (TMJD)
temporomaxillary
temporo-occipital
temporoparietal
    aphasia, t.
temporopontile
temporospatial
temporosphenoid
temporozygomatic
tenacious sputum
tenacity
tenaculum
tendon
    stapedius t.
tenebric vertigo
Tennison
    hairlip repair, T.
Tennison-Randall cleft lip repair
TENS (transcutaneous electrical nerve
    stimulation)
tension band wiring

tensor
    fascia, t.
    tympani, t.
    vela palatini, t.
tent
    croup t.
    mist t.
    oxygen t.
    steam t.
tentorial
tentorium
terfenadine
terminal
    abutment, t.
    loop, t.
terpin hydrate
Terpinol
tertiary dentin
Tessalon Perles
Tessier
    classification, T.
    craniofacial cleft, T.
    craniofacial operation, T.
    facial dysostosis operation, T.
tetanic
tetaniform
tetanigenous
tetanoid
tetanometer
tetanus
    toxin, t.
    toxoid, t.
tetany
Thal
    esophageal stricture repair, T.
    esophagogastrostomy, T.
    hiatal hernia repair, T.
thecodont
Theimich lip sign
Theobald
    lacrimal dilator, T.
    sinus probe, T.
Theolair
theophylline
Theovent
Therapybird

thermolaryngoscope
Thiersch
    graft, T.
    operation, T.
thimble
thinned down
third
    molar, t.
    pharyngeal pouch, t.
    tonsil, t.
13-q deletion syndrome
Thom flap laryngeal reconstruction
Thompson
    abscess, T.
    adenoid punch, T.
    antral rasp, T.
    frontal sinus raspatory, T.
    line, T.
    procedure, T.
thoracotomy
Thorazine
Thornell microlaryngoscopy
Thornwald
    antral drill, T.
    antral trephine, T.
    perforator, T.
    trephine, T.
Thornwaldt disease
thread-elastic ligation
three-day measles
three-quarter crown
threshold
throat
    culture, t.
    flora, t.
    forceps, t.
    irrigation tube, t.
    pack, t.
    scissors, t.
    smear, t.
    spray, t.
    swab, t.
    washings, t.
throb
throbbing pain
thrombin

thrombin *(continued)*
    -soaked Gelfoam, t.
Thrombinar
thrombolytic
thrombophlebitic
thrombophlebitis
thrombosis
    cavernous sinus t.
Thrombostat
thrush
thumb-sucker
thumb-sucking
thunderclap headache
thymic asthma
Thymoliodide powder
thyroarytenoideus muscle
thyroepiglotticus muscle
thyroglossal
    duct, t.
    duct cyst, t.
    sinus, t.
thyrohoid
    arch, t.
    bursa, t.
thyrohyoideus
thyroadenitis
thyroarytenoid
thyroarytenoideus
thyrochondrotomy
thyrocricotomy
thyroepiglottic
thyroepiglotticus
thyroepiglottideus
thyrofissure
thyroglossal
    cyst, t.
    duct, t.
    nerve, t.
thyrohyal
thyrohyoid
thyroid
    aberrant t.
    accessory t.
    ectopic t.
    intrathoracic t.
    lingual t.

thyroid *(continued)*
    retrosternal t.
    substernal t.
thyroid axis
thyroid cachexia
thyroid cartilage
thyroid collar
thyroid crisis
thyroid diverticulum
thyroid drain
thyroid eminence
thyroid extract
thyroid function test
thyroid gland
thyroid imaging
thyroid insufficiency
thyroid isthmectomy
thyroid isthmus
thyroid lobe
thyroid notch
thyroid red line
thyroid scan
thyroid scintigram
thyroid sonogram
thyroid stimulating hormone (TSH)
thyroid storm
thyroid uptake
thyroidea
    accessoria, t.
    ima, t.
thyroidectomize
thyroidectomy
    medical t.
thyroiditis
    acute t.
    autoimmune t.
    chronic t.
    chronic fibrous t.
    chronic lymphadenoid t.
    chronic lymphocytic t.
    de Quervain t.
    giant cell t.
    giant follicular t.
    granulomatous t.
    Hashimoto t.
    invasive t.

thyroiditis *(continued)*
  ligneous t.
  lymphocytic t.
  lymphoid t.
  pseudotuberculous t.
  Riedel t.
  subacute granulomatous t.
  subacute lymphocytic t.
  woody t.
thyroidization
thyroidorrhaphy
thyroidotomy
thyrointoxication
thyrolaryngeal
  fascia, t.
thyrolingual
  duct, t.
  trunk, t.
thyromegaly
thyroparathyroidectomy
thyropathy
thyropharyngeal muscle
thyroprival
thyroprivia
thyrotomy
thyrotoxic
  goiter, t.
  storm, t.
thyrotoxicosis
  factitia, t.
thyrotropic
thyroxin
thyroxine
tic
  convulsive t.
  de sommeil, t.
  douloureaux, t.
  facial t.
  gesticulatory t.
  habit t.
  laryngeal t.
  local t.
  mimic t.
  motor t.
  progressive choreic t.
  rotatoire, t.

tic *(continued)*
  spasmodic t.
Tieck nasal speculum
tie-over bolus dressing
tight asthmatic
Tilden method
timber tongue
tin foil
tinnitus
  aurium, t.
  clicking t.
  Leudet t.
  nervous t.
  nonvibratory t.
  objective t.
  vibratory t.
tinted denture base
tip
  deformity, t.
  dressing, t.
  graft, t.
  -plasty, t.
tipping
tiqueur
tissue
  bank, t.
  conduction, t.
  expander, t.
  graft, t.
titanium
  dioxide, t.
  graft, t.
  miniplate, t.
  plate, t.
  screw, t.
Titterington position
titillation
titubation
  lingual t.
Titus tongue depressor
Tivnen tonsil-seizing forceps
TM (temporomandibular or tympanic membrane)
TMJ (temporomandibular joint)
  ankylosis, T.
  ganglion, T.

TMJ (temporomandibular joint) *(continued)*
    splint, T.
TMJD (temporomandibular joint dysfunction)
TNM (tumor, nodes, metastasis) classification
TNS (transcutaneous nerve stimulator)
Tobey
    ear forceps, T.
    rongeur, T.
Tobey-Ayer test
Tobold
    knife, T.
    laryngeal forceps, T.
toddy
toilette
tolu balsam
Tomes
    fiber, T.
    fibril, T.
    granular layer, T.
    process, T.
tomolaryngography
tone
    deafness, t.
    decay, t.
    decay test, t. (TDT)
tongs
    skull t.
tongue
    adherent t.
    amyloid t.
    antibiotic t.
    baked t.
    bald t.
    beefy t.
    bifid t.
    black t.
    black hairy t.
    burning t.
    cardinal t.
    cerebriform t.
    choreic t.
    cleft t.
    coated t.

tongue *(continued)*
    cobblestone t.
    crocodile t.
    Crombie t.
    dotted t.
    double t.
    dry t.
    earthy t.
    encrusted t.
    fern leaf t.
    filmy t.
    fissured t.
    flat t.
    forked t.
    furred t.
    furry t.
    furrowed t.
    geographic t.
    grooved t.
    hairy t.
    lobulated t.
    magenta t.
    mappy t.
    parrot t.
    phossy t.
    plicated t.
    raspberry t.
    red strawberry t.
    Sandwith bald t.
    scrotal t.
    smokers' t.
    smooth t.
    split t.
    stippled t.
    strawberry t.
    sulcated t.
    timber t.
    trifid t.
    trombone t.
    white t.
    white strawberry t.
    wooden t.
    wrinkled t.
tongue blade
tongue bone
tongue depressor

tongue flap
tongue forceps
tongue phenomen
tongue protrusion
tongue retractor blade
tongue retrusion
tongue-seizing forceps
tongue suture
tongue-swallowing
tongue thrust
tongue-tie
tongue traction
tonsil
    adenoid t.
    buried t.
    cerebellar t.
    cryptic t.
    eustachian t.
    faucial t.
    Gerlach t.
    hypertrophied t.
    kissing t's.
    lingual t.
    Luschka t.
    nasal t.
    palatine t.
    pharyngeal t.
    submerged t.
    third t.
    torus tubarius, t. of
    tubal t's
tonsil caliper
tonsil clamp
tonsil compressor
tonsil dissector
tonsil electrode
tonsil elevator
tonsil enucleator
tonsil expressor
tonsil forceps
tonsil guillotine
tonsil hemostat
tonsil hook
tonsil knife
tonsil-ligating forceps
tonsil needle
tonsil position
tonsil punch
tonsil retractor
tonsil scissors
tonsil screw
tonsil-seizing forceps
tonsil separator
tonsil slitter
tonsil snare
tonsil sponge
tonsil spreader
tonsil suction tip
tonsil suture hook
tonsil suture needle
tonsil syringe
tonsil tampon
tonsilla (pl. tonsillae)
    adenoidea, t.
    lingualis, t.
    palatina, t.
    pharyngealis, t.
    tubaria, t.
tonsillae (pl. of tonsilla)
tonsillar
    abscess, t.
    area, t.
    calculus, t.
    calipers, t.
    capsule, t.
    compressor, t.
    crypts, t.
    electrode, t.
    elevator, t.
    enucleator, t.
    expressor, t.
    exudate, t.
    forceps, t.
    fossa, t.
    hernia, t.
    invasive tongue lesion, t.
    pad, t.
    pillar, t.
    ring, t.
    sinus, t.
    tag, t.
tonsillectome

tonsillectomy
    adenoidectomy, t. and (T&A)
tonsillith
tonsillitic
tonsillitis
    acute t.
    caseous t.
    catarrhal t.
    diphtherial t.
    erythematous t.
    exudative t.
    follicular t.
    herpetic t.
    lacunar t.
    lenta, t.
    lingual t.
    mycotic t.
    parenchymatous t.
    preglottic t.
    pustular t.
    streptococcal t.
    superficial t.
    suppurative t.
    Vincent t.
tonsilloadenoidectomy
tonsillohemisporosis
tonsillolith
tonsillomoniliasis
tonsillomycosis
tonsillo-oidiosis
tonsillopathy
tonsilloscope
tonsilloscopy
tonsillotome
tonsillotomy
tonsillotyphoid
tonsolith
tooth
    abutment t.
    accessional t.
    anatomic t.
    ankylosed t.
    anterior t.
    artificial t.
    auditory t. of Huschka
    axis, t. of

tooth *(continued)*
    baby t.
    bicuspid t.
    buccal t.
    canine t.
    capped t.
    cheek t.
    conical t.
    connate t.
    corner t.
    cross-bite t.
    cross-pin t.
    cuspid t.
    cuspless t.
    decayed t.
    deciduous t.
    diatoric t.
    drifting t.
    embedded t.
    epistropheus, t. of
    erupted t.
    eye t.
    filled t.
    floating t.
    Fournier t.
    fractured t.
    fused t.
    geminate t.
    Goslee t.
    graft t.
    hag t.
    hair t.
    Horner t.
    Hutchinson t.
    impacted t.
    implantation t.
    implanted t.
    incisor t.
    labial t.
    lion's t.
    malacotic t.
    malposed t.
    mandibular t.
    maxillary t.
    metal insert t.
    milk t.

tooth *(continued)*
   mobile t.
   molar t.
   Moon t.
   morsal t.
   mottled t.
   mulberry t.
   natal t.
   neonatal t.
   nonanatomic t.
   nonvital t.
   peg t.
   peg-shaped t.
   permanent t.
   pink t. of Mummery
   pinless t.
   posterior t.
   predeciduous t.
   premature t.
   premolar t.
   primary t.
   pulpless t.
   rake t.
   reimplanted t.
   retruded t.
   rootless t.
   sclerotic t.
   screwdriver t.
   secondary t.
   shell t.
   snaggle t.
   stained t.
   stomach t.
   straight-pin t.
   submerged t.
   succedaneous t.
   successional t.
   superior t.
   supernumerary t.
   supplemental t.
   supporting structure t.
   temporary t.
   transplantation t.
   tube t.
   Turner t.
   unerupted t.

tooth *(continued)*
   vital t.
   wandering t.
   wisdom t.
   yellow t.
   zero degree t.
tooth abrasion
tooth abscess
tooth absence
tooth anchoring
tooth angles
tooth attrition
tooth band
tooth banding
tooth bonding
tooth-borne
tooth bud
tooth calcification
tooth cap
tooth crypt
tooth bud
tooth decay
tooth dwarfism
tooth elevator
tooth erosion
tooth-extracting forceps
tooth extraction
tooth fusion
tooth gemination
tooth germ
tooth giantism
tooth hood
tooth implantation
tooth ligation
tooth maturation
tooth powder
tooth pulp
tooth rash
tooth reimplantation
tooth repair
tooth root
tooth socket
tooth transplantation
toothache
toothbrush
   trauma, t.

toothpaste
tophi (pl. of tophus)
   gouty t.
tophus (pl. tophi)
topical
   cocaine, t.
   decongestant, t.
   spray, t.
Topinard
   angle, T.
   line, T.
Topostasine
torcular Herophili
Torek esophagectomy
tori (pl. of torus)
Tornwaldt
   abscess, T.
   bursa, T.
   bursitis, T.
   cyst, t.
TORP (total ossicular replacement prosthesis)
torque
torqued
torquing
   key, t.
   tooth, t. of
torsed
torsion
   test, t.
torsiversion
torticollar
torticollis
   atlanto-epistrophealis, t.
   congenital t.
   dermatogenic t.
   fixed t.
   hysteric t.
   hysterical t.
   intermittent t.
   labyrinthine t.
   mental t.
   myogenic t.
   nasopharyngiene, t.
   neurogenic t.
   ocular t.

torticollis *(continued)*
   reflex t.
   rheumatic t.
   rheumatoid t.
   spasmodic t.
   spurious t.
   symptomatic t.
tortua facies
tortuous
   esophagus, t.
   root canal, t.
torus (pl. tori)
   frontalis, t.
   levatorius, t.
   mandibulae, t.
   mandibularis, t.
   occipitalis, t.
   palatinus, t.
   tubarius, t.
total
   cheek mucosa defect, t.
   laryngectomy, t.
   ossicular replacement prosthesis, t. (TORP)
Tote-A-Neb nebulizer
Toti operation
Toupet esophageal fundoplication
Tourette syndrome
touretter
Tourtual canal
Towne projection
toxic
   appearance, t.
   deafness, t.
   goiter, t.
Toynbee
   ear speculum, T.
   law, T.
   ligament, T.
   maneuver, T.
   otoscope, T.
   speculum, T.
trachea (pl. tracheae)
   scabbard t.
tracheae (pl. of trachea)
tracheaectasy

tracheal
- amyloidosis, t.
- aspirate, t.
- aspiration, t.
- atresia, t.
- band, t.
- bifurcation nodes, t.
- bistoury, t.
- bougie, t.
- bronchus, t.
- button, t.
- cannula, t.
- cartilage, t.
- catheter, t.
- compression, t.
- deviation, t.
- dilatation, t.
- dilation, t.
- dilator, t.
- diverticulosis, t.
- diverticulum, t.
- duplication, t.
- fistula, t.
- forceps, t.
- fracture, t.
- hemostat, t.
- hook, t.
- intubation, t.
- knife, t.
- lavage, t.
- lymph nodes, t.
- mucus, t.
- muscle, t.
- obstruction, t.
- perforation, t.
- rales, t.
- retractor, t.
- rings, t.
- scissors, t.
- secretions, t.
- shift, t.
- spill, t.
- stenosis, t.
- stump, t.
- suction tube, t.
- tampon, t.

tracheal *(continued)*
- tenaculum, t.
- tone, t.
- tree, t.
- tube, t.
- tug, t.
- web, t.

trachealgia
trachealis
tracheitis
trachelagra
trachelematoma
trachelism
trachelismus
trachelocyllosis
trachelodynia
trachelology
trachelomastoid
trachelomyitis
tracheloschisis
tracheoaerocele
tracheobronchial
- lavage, t.
- lymph nodes, t.
- suction tube, t.
- toilette, t.
- tree, t.
- tuberculosis, t.

tracheobronchitis
tracheobronchomegaly
tracheobronchoscopy
tracheocannula
tracheocele
tracheocricotomy
tracheoesophageal (TE)
- fistula, t. (TEF)
- septum, t.
- shunt, t.

tracheofissure
tracheofistulization
tracheogenic
tracheogram
tracheography
tracheolaryngeal
tracheolaryngotomy
tracheomalacia

tracheomegaly
tracheopathia
   osteoplastica, t.
tracheopathy
tracheopharyngeal
tracheophonesis
tracheophony
tracheoplasty
tracheopyosis
tracheorrhagia
tracheorrhaphy
tracheoschisis
tracheoscope
tracheoscopic
tracheoscopy
   peroral t.
tracheostenosis
tracheostoma
tracheostome
tracheostomize
tracheostomy
   aerosol mask, t.
   button, t.
   cannula, t.
   care, t.
   cuff, t.
   hook, t.
   scissors, t.
   stoma, t.
   trocar, t.
   tube, t.
tracheotome
tracheotomic bistoury
tracheotomize
tracheotomy
   cannula, t.
   hook, t.
   set, t.
   tube, t.
trachitis
Trach-Mist
Trach-Talk
trachoma (pl. trachomata)
   vocal bands, t. of
trachomata (pl. of trachoma)
trachomatous

trachyphonia
traction
   elastic t.
   external t.
   intermaxillary t.
   internal t.
   maxillomandibular t.
   tongue t.
traction diverticulum
tragal
tragi (pl. of tragus)
tragion
tragophony
tragus (pl. tragi)
Trainor-Nida technique
transantral
transcanal
transcolumellar
   flying-bird incision, t.
transconjunctival
transcortical aphasia
transcricothyroid
transcutaneous
   electrical nerve stimulation, t. (TENS)
   nerve stimulator, t. (TCNS or TNS)
Transderm-Scop
transesophageal
   echocardiography, t.
   ligation of varices, t.
   probe, t.
transethmoidal
   hypophysectomy, t.
   sphenoidotomy, t.
transfacial
transfer coping
transfixion suture
transglottic
transglottis
transillumination
transisthmian
transitional denture
transmeatal
transmission
   deafness, t.
   hearing loss, t.
transnasal

transnasal *(continued)*
    drain, t.
    sphenoidotomy, t.
transnasally
transoral
    approach, t.
    projection, t.
transorbital
transosseous implant
transosteal implant
transpalatal
transposition flap
transseptal
transsphenoidal
    hypophysectomy, t.
    resection, t.
transtracheal
    aspiration, t.
transtympanic
    neurectomy, t.
transudate
transudation
transverse horizontal vermilionectomy
trapezius osteomyocutaneous flap
trauma
    occlusal t.
    toothbrush t.
traumatic
    aphasia, t.
    apnea, t.
    deafness, t.
traumatogenic
    occlusion, t.
    pulpal occlusion, t.
Trauner lingual sulcus extension
Trautmann triangle
tray
    dental t.
    impression t.
Treacher Collins syndrome
Treacher Collins-Franceschetti syndrome
tree
    bronchial t.
    tracheobronchial t.
trench mouth
Trendelenburg position

trephination
trephine
trephinement
trephining
Tresilian sign
triad
trial base
triamcinolone acetonide dental paste
triangle
triangular
    cartilage of nose, t.
    eminence, t.
trichloroacetic acid
trichoglossia
trichorhinopharyngeal
    sign, t.
    syndrome, t.
tricuspid tooth
trifacial
    neuralgia, t.
trifid tongue
trigeminal
    cough, t.
    mandibular division, t.
    maxillary division, t.
    nerve, t.
    neuralgia, t.
    sphenopalatine ganglion, t.
    submaxillary ganglion, t.
trigonal
trigone
Trimadeau sign
Tri-Met apnea monitor
trimmer
    gingival margin t.
    model t.
Tripier technique
triple antibiotics
tripod fracture
tripoli
triquetral cartilage
trismic
trisomic
trisomy
trismus
    nascentium, t.

triticeous
  cartilage, t.
triturate
trituration
triturator
trocar
troche
trochiscus
trochlea (pl. trochleae)
trochleae (pl. of trochlea)
trochlear
trochleariform
trochlearis
Troeltsch
  ear forceps, T.
  ear speculum, T.
  recesses, T.
Trolard plexus
trombone tremor of tongue
tromophonia
trophoneurosis
  facial t.
tropical ear
trough
  gingival t.
Trousseau-Jackson
  esophageal dilator, T.
  tracheal dilator, T.
Troutman
  mastoid chisel, T.
  mastoid gouge, T.
Tru-Arc trachea tube
Truc technique
true
  anodontia, t.
  aphasia, t.
  asthma, t.
  cementoma, t.
  vertigo, t.
  vocal cords, t. (TVC)
try-in wax
TSH (thyroid stimulating hormone)
T-tube (tympanostomy tube)
tuba (pl. tubae)
  acustica, t.
  auditiva, t.

tuba (pl. tubae) *(continued)*
  auditoria, t.
tubae (pl. of tuba)
tubal
  block, t.
  canal, t.
  cartilage, t.
  ear, t.
  tonsil, t.
tube
  air t.
  auditory t.
  Bouchut t's
  buccal t.
  Celestin t.
  end t.
  endobronchial t.
  endotracheal t.
  esophageal t.
  eustachian t.
  horizontal t.
  intubation t.
  Levin t.
  nasogastric t.
  otopharyngeal t.
  pharyngotympanic t.
  Ruysch t.
  Sengstaken-Blakemore t.
  Souttar t.
  sputum t.
  T t.
  tracheostomy t.
  tracheotomy t.
tube flap
tube pedicle
tube teeth
tubed flap
Tube-Lok tracheotomy dressing
tuber (pl. tubera)
tubera (pl. of tuber)
tubercle
  acoustic t.
  amygdaloid t. of Schwalbe
  articular t.
  auditory t.
  auricular t.

tubercle *(continued)*
   condyloid t.
   darwinian t.
   dental t.
   epiglottic t.
   genial t.
   His t.
   jugular t.
   lacrimal t.
   lateral orbital t.
   lateral palpebral t.
   marginal t. of zygomatic bone
   mental t.
   Morgagni t.
   olfactory t.
   pharyngeal t.
   pterygoid t.
   root of zygoma, t. of
   sella turcica, t. of
   thyroid t.
   upper lip, t. of
   Whitnall t.
   zygomatic t.
tuberculosis
tuberculous gingivitis
tuberosity
   malar t.
   masseteric t.
   maxillary t.
   pterygoid t. of mandible
   pyramidal t. of palatine bone
tubopharyngeal ligament of Rauber
tuboplasty
tuborrhea
tubotorsion
tubotympanal
tubotympanic
   canal, t.
   recess, t.
tubotympanum
Tucker
   bougie, T.
   bronchoscope, T.
   dilator, T.
   esophagoscope, T.
   forceps, T.

Tucker *(continued)*
   laryngoscope, T.
   spray, T.
Tucker-McLane forceps
Tuebingen-type implant
tuft
   enamel t.
tugging
   tracheal t.
Tulevec lacrimal cannula
tumbler flap
tumeur perlee
tuning fork
tunnel procedure
   Corti, t. of
   procedure, t.
turbid fluid
turbinal
   crest, t.
turbinate
   inferior t.
   middle t.
   nasal t.
   superior t.
turbinate bone
turbinate electrode
turbinate firing
turbinate firing needle
turbinated
turbinectomy
turbinotome
turbinotomy
turboplasty
Turck trachoma
turkey gobbler neck
Turner
   mosaicism, T.
   syndrome, T.
   tooth, T.
Tuss-Ade
tussal
Tussend
tussicula
tussicular
tussiculation
tussigenic

tussis
  convulsiva, t.
  stomachalis t.
tussive
  fremitus, t.
  squeeze, t.
  syncope, t.
Tuss-Ornade
TVC (true vocal cord)
Tweed triangle
  twelfth-year molar, t.
twin wire appliance
Twisk needleholder
Tydings
  forceps, T.
  knife, T.
  snare, T.
  tonsillectome, T.
Tydings-Lakeside forceps
Tygon esophageal prosthesis
tympanal
tympanectomy
tympanic
  annulus, t.
  antrum, t.
  bone, t.
  canal, t.
  canaliculus, t.
  cavity, t.
  lip, t.
  membrane, t. (TM)
  nerve, t.
  notch, t.
  orifice, t.
  plate, t.
  plexus, t.
  ring, t.
  scute, t.
  sinus, t.
  sulcus, t.
tympanitis
tympanocentesis
tympanocervical
  abscess, t.
tympanichord
tympanichordal

tympanicity
tympanitic
tympanitis
tympanoacryloplasty
tympanocentesis
tympanoeustachian
tympanogram
tympanography
tympanohyal
tympanolabyrinthopexy
tympanomalleal
tympanomandibular
  cartilage, t.
tympanomastoid
  abscess, t.
  cavity, t.
  fissure, t.
tympanomastoidectomy
tympanomastoiditis
tympanomeatal
  flap, t.
tympanometry
tympano-ossicular
tympanophonia
tympanoplastic
  knife, t.
tympanoplasty (types I, II, III, IV, and V)
tympanosclerosis
tympanosclerotic
tympanoscope
Tympan-O-Scope
tympanoscopy
tympanosquamosal
tympanosquamous
tympanostapedial
tympanostomy
  tube, t. (T-tube)
  ventilation tube, t.
tympanosympathectomy
tympanotemporal
tympanotomy
  flap, t.
tympanum
  perforator, t.
tympany
typodont

U

UAO (upper airway obstruction)
Ueckermann cricothyroid trocar
Ueckermann-Denker trocar
Ueno procedure
UES (upper esophageal sphincter)
UG (ultrasound-guided)
UGFNAB (ultrasound-guided fine-needle aspiration biopsy)
ulaganactesis
ulalgia
ulatrophia
ulatrophy
   afunctional u.
   atrophic u.
   calcic u.
   ischemic u.
   traumatic u.
ulcer
   aphthous u.
   Barrett u.
   chicle u.
   chiclero u.
   Cushing-Rokitansky u.
   follicular u.
   peptic u.
   Rokitansky-Cushing u.
   soft u.
   sublingual u.
ulcerated
   plaque, u.
   tooth, u.
ulceration
   Daguet, u. of
ulcerative
   lesion, u.
   plaque, u.
ulceromembranous
   gingivitis, u.
   tonsillitis, u.
ulectomy
ulitis
   interstitial u.
Ulloa technique

Ullrich-Feichtiger syndrome
Ullrich-Turner syndrome
ulocace
ulocarcinoma
uloglossitis
uloncus
ulorrhagia
ulorrhea
ulotomy
ulotripsis
ultimobranchial bodies
ultrasonic
   nebulizer, u.
   scaler, u.
   scaling, u.
ultrasonogram
ultrasonography
ultrasound
   -guided, u. (UG)
   -guided fine-needle aspiration biopsy, u. (UGFNAB)
umbo (pl. umbones)
   tympanic membrane, u. of
umbonate
umbones (pl. of umbo)
U-Mid/02 Jet Set
unattached gingiva
unciform
   fasciculus, u.
   process, u.
uncinate
   bodies of Russell, u.
   fits, u.
   process, u.
uncinatum
uncinectomy
undercut
underhung bite
undermine
undermining
undulatory nystagmus
Unger adenoid pressure roller
uniaural

unicuspid
unicuspidate
unilateral nystagmus
universal appliance
Universal
    antral punch, U.
    esophagoscope, U.
    handle with nasal-cutting tips, U.
unroof
unroofed
unroofing
upbiting
    forceps, u.
    scissors, u.
Updegraff cleft palate needle
updraft
upper
    airway obstruction, u. (UAO)
    esophageal sphincter, u. (UES)
    esophagoscope, u.
    esophagus, u.
    jaw, u.
    respiratory, u. (UR)
    respiratory infection, u. (URI)
    respiratory tract, u.
UPPP (uvulopalatopharyngoplasty)
uprighting
    spring, u.
uptake
    T-4 u.
    thyroid u.
UR (upper respiratory)
uranischochasma
uraniscolalia
uranisconitis
uraniscoplasty
uraniscorrhaphy
uraniscus
uranoplasty
uranoplegia
uranorrhaphy
uranoschisis
uranoschism
uranostaphyloplasty
uranostaphylorrhaphy
uranostaphyloschisis
unerupted teeth
URI (upper respiratory infection)
urogastrone
urticaria
urticarial
Usher disease
uterine cough
utility wax
utricle
utriculi (pl. of utriculus)
utriculitis
utriculosaccular
    canal, u.
    duct, u.
utriculus (pl. utriculi)
uveoneuraxitis
uveoparotid
uvula
    fissa, u.
    palatina, u.
    palatine u.
uvular
    cleft, u.
uvularis
uvulatomy
uvulectomy
uvulitis
uvulopalatine
uvulopalatopharyngoplasty (UPPP)
uvulopalatoplasty
uvulopharyngeal
uvulopharyngeus
uvulopharyngoplasty
uvuloplasty
uvuloptosis
uvulotome
uvulotomy

V

VACTERL (vertebral, anal, cardiac, tracheal, esophageal, renal, limb)
vacuum headache
vaginal throat pack
vagoglossopharyngeal
vagolysis
vagus nerve
Valentin
   ganglion, V.
   pseudoganglion, V.
vallecula (valleculae)
   epiglottica, v.
valleculae
vallecular
   dysphagia, v.
   pouch, v.
   sign, v.
Valsalva
   ligaments, V.
   maneuver, V.
   sinus, v.
valsalva'd
Van Alyea
   antral cannula, V.
   antral trocar, V.
   tube, V.
Vancenase inhaler
van der Hoeve syndrome
Van der Woude syndrome
Van Millingen
   eyelid repair technique, V.
   graft, V.
Van Osdel
   antral wash bottle, V.
   guillotine, V.
   tonsillar enucleator, V.
   tonsillar knife, V.
   tonsillectome, V.
Van Struycken
   nasal forceps, V.
   nasal punch, V.
vapor
vaporarium

vaporization
vaporize
vaporizer
vapotherapy
variceal
   hemorrhage, v.
   sclerosing procedure, v.
varicella
   zoster, v. (VZ)
   zoster virus, v. (VZV)
varices (pl. of varix)
   esophageal v.
varicosity
varix (pl. varices)
   esophageal v.
vasa
   auris internae, v.
vascular
   deafness, v.
   ring, v.
vasoconstriction
vasoconstrictor
vasodentin
vasomotor
   rhinitis, v.
vasovagal syncope
Vater duct
VATER (vertebral defects, imperforate anus, tracheoesophageal fistula, radial, ray, or renal anomaly)
vault
   cartilaginous v.
   nasal v.
   pharynx, v. of
Veau
   cleft lip repair, V.
   elevator, V.
   palatoplasty, V.
   straight-line closure, V.
Veau-Axhausen procedure
Veau-Wardill
   palatal push-back, V.
   palatoplasty, V.

Veau-Wardill-Kilner cleft palate repair
vector
vegetal bronchitis
vein of Galen
vela (pl. of velum)
velar
velolaryngeal
    endoscopy, v.
velopharyngeal
    insufficiency, v.
    portal, v.
velum (pl. vela)
    artificial v.
    Baker v.
    palatinum, v.
veneer crown
venereal collar
ventilate
ventilating
    tube, v.
ventilation
    bronchoscope, v.
    tube, v.
ventilatory
    assistance, v.
Venti-mask
Ventolin
ventricular band
ventriculocordotomy
Ventrol Levin tube
Venturi mask
verbal aphasia
Verga lacrimal groove
Verhoeff technique
vermilion
    border, v.
    margin, v.
    surface of lip, v.
vermilionectomy
Vernet syndrome
vertical
    nystagmus, v.
    vertigo, v.
verticosubmental
vertiginous
vertigo

vertigo *(continued)*
    ab stomacho laeso, v.
    alternobaric v.
    angiopathic v.
    apoplectic v.
    arteriosclerotic v.
    auditory v.
    aural v.
    benign paroxysmal positional v.
    cardiac v.
    cardiovascular v.
    central v.
    cerebral v.
    disabling positional v.
    encephalic v.
    endemic paralytic v.
    epidemic v.
    epileptic v.
    essential v.
    galvanic v.
    gastric v.
    height v.
    hysterical v.
    labyrinthine v.
    laryngeal v.
    lateral v.
    lithemic v.
    mechanical v.
    neurasthenic v.
    nocturnal v.
    objective v.
    ocular v.
    organic v.
    paralyzing v.
    peripheral v.
    pilot's v.
    positional v.
    postural v.
    pressure v.
    primary v.
    residual v.
    riders' v.
    rotary v.
    rotatory v.
    sham-movement v.
    special sense v.

vertigo *(continued)*
    stomachal v.
    subjective v.
    systematic v.
    tenebric v.
    toxemic v.
    toxic v.
    vertical v.
    vestibular v.
    villous v.
    voltaic v.
verrucous
    carcinoma, v.
    lesion, v.
vertical
    augmentation genioplasty, v.
    overlap, v.
Verweys technique
vesicular
    bronchitis, v.
    pharyngitis, v.
    rash, v.
vestibula (pl. of vestibulum)
vestibular
    aqueduct, v.
    ataxia, v.
    canal, v.
    clamp, v.
    crest, v.
    labyrinth, v.
    ligament, v.
    nerve, v.
    neuronitis, v.
    nystagmus, v.
    osteotomy, v.
    reflex, v.
    root, v.
    screen, v.
    system, v.
    vertigo, v.
    window, v.
vestibule
    buccal v.
    ear, v. of
    inner ear, v. of
    internal ear, v. of

vestibule *(continued)*
    labial v.
    labyrinth, v. of
    larynx, v. of
    mouth, v. of
    nasal cavity, v. of
    nose, v. of
    pharynx, v. of
vestibulocochlear
vestibulocochlearis
vestibuloequilibratory
vestibulogenic
vestibulo-ocular
vestibuloplasty
vestibulotomy
vestibulum (pl. vestibula)
    auris, v.
    glottidis, v.
    laryngis, v.
    nasi, v.
    oris, v.
vestige
vestigial nodule
via
vibrating line
vibration
vibratory
    nystagmus, v.
    sense, v.
vibrissa (pl. vibrissae)
vibrissae (pl. of vibrissa)
vibromasseur
vibrometer
Vickers hardness test
Vicq d'Azyr laryngeal procedure
Victorian collar dressing
vidian
    artery, v.
    canal, v.
    nerve, v.
    neuralgia, v.
Vienna nasal speculum
Vieussen
    annulus, V.
Villaret syndrome
villous vertigo

Vim tonsil syringe
Vincent
  angina, V.
  gingivitis, V.
  infection, V.
  stomatitis, V.
  tonsillitis, V.
Vinson syndrome
viral
  exanthem, v.
  upper respiratory infection, v.
  URI, v.
Virchow
  angle, V.
  line, V.
viscid
viscosity
viscous
visor flap
visual
  aphasia, v.
  axis, v.
  hearing, v.
  nystagmus, v.
visuoauditory
visuosensory
vital tooth
Vitalog monitor
Vitallium
  glenoid fossa prosthesis, V.
  ramus, V.
vitamin C
Vivonex Moss tube
Vladimiroff operation
VLIA (virus-like infectious agent)
V.M. & Co. mastoid curette
vocal
  cords, v.
  cord stripping, v.
  cordectomy, v.
  cordotomy, v.
  fold, v.
  fremitus, v.
  ligament, v.
  lips, v.
  muscle, v.

vocal *(continued)*
  nodule, v.
  process, v.
  resonance, v.
  signs, v.
vocalis muscle
Vogel
  adenoid curette, V.
  infant adenoid curette, V.
  otoplasty, V.
Vogt
  angle, V.
  syndrome, V.
Vogt-Koyanagi syndrome
voice
  amphoric v.
  cavernous v.
  double v.
  eunuchoid v.
  whispered v.
voice box
voice button
voice prosthesis
voice rest
voice restoration
voiceprint
voices
voix
  de polichinelle, v.
voltaic vertigo
Voltolini
  disease, V.
  ear tube, V.
  septum speculum, V.
voluntary nystagmus
vomer
  bone, v.
  ridge, v.
vomerine
  canal, v.
  groove, v.
  plate, v.
  spur, v.
vomerobasilar
  canal, v.
vomeronasal

vomeronasal *(continued)*
   cartilage, v.
   organs of Jacobson, v.
vomerorostral canal
vomerovaginal canal
von Bezold abscess
von Blaskovics-Doyen technique
von Graefe sign
von Langenbeck
   bipedicle mucoperiosteal flap, v.
   cleft lip repair, v.
von Recklinghausen disease
von Willebrand disease
VoSol HC
VoSol otic
vox
   abscissa, v.
   capitus, v.

vox *(continued)*
   cholerica, v.
   rauca, v.
V-shaped arch
vulcanite
   bur, v.
   dental plate, v.
V-Vac suction apparatus
V-Y
   advancement flap, V.
   palatoplasty, V.
   push-back cleft palate repair, V.
   repair of cheek defect, V.
   retroposition cleft palate repair, V.
V-Z
   advancement in buccal sulcus, V.
VZ (varicella zoster)
VZV (varicella-zoster virus)

Additional entries

W

Waardenburg syndrome
Wader and Andrews tongue depressor
Wagener ear hook
Wagner
   antrum punch, W.
   laryngeal brush, W.
   skull resection, W.
waisting
Waldeyer
   gland, W.
   odontoblasts, W.
   ring, W.
   tonsillar ring, W.
Walker
   appliance, W.
   dissector, W.
   tonsil suction dissector, W.
Wallenberg syndrome
Walsham
   nasal forceps, W.
   septum-straightening forceps, W.
Walther duct
Walton ear knife
waltzed flap
waltzing
wandering
   goiter, w.
   rash, w.
   tooth, w.
Wangensteen tube
Wardill palatoplasty
Wardill-Kilner
   cleft palate repair, W.
   four-flap technique, W.
Waring tonsil suction tube
warm nodule
Warthin tumor
Warthin-Finkeldy cells
washings
   bronchial w.
   nasopharyngeal w.
wasp-waist laryngoscope
water

water *(continued)*
   brash, w.
   choke, w.
   -gurgle test, w.
   -infusion esophageal manometry catheter, w.
   pick, w.
Water-Pik
Waterhouse-Friderichsen syndrome
Waterman bronchoscope
Waters
   position, W.
   view, W.
watery discharge
Watson tonsil-seizing forceps
Watson-Williams
   ethmoidal punch, W.
   ethmoid-biting forceps, W.
   frontal sinus rasp, W.
   nasal forceps, W.
   nasal polypus, W.
   sinus rasp, W.
   sinus raspatory, W.
wax
   baseplate w.
   bone w.
   boxing w.
   burnout w.
   casting w.
   dental w.
   inlay w.
   pattern w.
wax bite
wax carver
waxing
waxing die
waxing-up
weak contact
Weaver sinus probe
web
   esophageal w.
   laryngeal w.
   neck, w. of

web *(continued)*
   tracheal w.
webbed neck
webbing
Weber
   glands, W.
   nasal douche, W.
   paralysis, W.
   test, W.
Webster
   cheiloplasty, W.
   needle holder, W.
Weck-cel sponge
Weder tongue depressor
Weder-Solenberger tonsillar pillar retractor
wedge elevator
weeping lesion
Weerda distending operating laryngoscope
Wegner granulomatosis
Weil
   basal layer, W.
   ear forceps, W.
   ethmoidal forceps, W.
   lacrimal cannula, W.
Weingartner ear forceps
Weir
   excision, W.
   incision, W.
   procedure, W.
Weisbach angle
Weisman ear curette
Weitlaner retractor
Welch-Allyn
   AudioScope, W.
   Kleenspec laryngoscope, W.
   laryngoscope, W.
   otoscope, W.
   probe, W.
   speculum, W.
   tube, W.
Wellaminski antrum perforator
Werb rhinostomy scissors
Wernicke
   aphasia, W.

Wernicke *(continued)*
   area, W.
Wesson mouth gag
West
   dacryocystorhinostomy, W.
   nasal-dressing forceps, W.
Westmacott nasal dressing forceps
wet
   cough, w.
   swallows, w.
Weyers oligodactyly syndrome
whalebone
   eustachian bougie, w.
   eustachian probe, w.
   filiform bougie, w.
Wharton duct
wheal
wheel
   carborundum w.
   diamond w.
   polishing w.
   wire w.
Wheeler technique
wheeze
wheezing
wheezy
whinolalia
whiplash
whirlybird stapes excavator
whisper
whispered
   bronchophony, w.
   pectoriloquy, w.
   voice test, w.
whistling face
   syndrome, w.
   -windmill vane hand syndrome, w.
white
   mouth, w.
   noise, w.
   strawberry tongue, w.
   tongue, w.
White
   forceps, W.
   mastoid rongeur, W.
   tonsil forceps, W.

White-Lillie tonsil forceps
White-Proud retractor
Whitehead
    deformity, W.
    mouth gag, W.
    radical glossectomy, W.
whitening
whiting
Whiting
    curette, W.
    rongeur, W.
    tonsillectome, W.
Whitnall tubercle
whoop
whooping cough
Wicherkiewicz eyelid repair
Wichmann
    asthma, W.
    syndrome, W.
wick
Wickwitz esophageal stricture
Widowitz sign
Wieder retractor
Wiener
    antral raspatory, W.
    eyelid repair, W.
    rasp, W.
    technique, W.
    Universal fronal antral rasp, W.
Wiener-Pierce
    antral rasp, W.
    antral trocar, W.
Wiener-Sauer intranasal tear-sac instruments
Wies lid fracturing technique
wild cherry
Wilde
    ear forceps, W.
    ethmoidal exenteration forceps, W.
    incision, W.
    nasal snare, W.
    punch, W.
    septal forceps, W.
Wilde-Blakesley ethmoidal forceps
Wilde-Bruening snare
Wildermuth ear

Williams
    ear perforator, W.
    elfin facies syndrome, W.
    lacrimal dilator, W.
    tonsil electrode, W.
    tracheal tone, W.
Willis paracusis
Willock respiratory jacket
window
    cochlear w.
    oval w.
    round w.
    vestibular w.
window crown
window operation
window rasp
window resection
windowing
windpipe
winged
    incisor, w.
    scapula, w.
winking
    -jaw syndrome, w.
    spasm, w.
Winkler disease
Winter
    arch bars, W.
    syndrome, W.
winter
    cold, w.
    cough, w.
wire
    arch w.
    ligature w.
    separating w.
    stainless steel w.
wire cutters
wire-fat ear prosthesis
wire loop stapes dilator
wire piston
wire stapes prosthesis
wire twisters
wire-wound endotracheal tube
wiring
    circumferential w.

wiring *(continued)*
   continuous loop w.
   craniofacial suspension w.
   Gilmer w.
   intermaxillary w.
   Ivy loop w.
   jaw, w. of
   perialveolar w.
   pyriform w.
   Stout w.
   teeth, w. of
Wis-Foregger laryngoscope
Wis-Hipple laryngoscope
wisdom tooth
Wistar pyramids
Woake saw
Wolf mouth gag
Wolf-Hirschhorn syndrome
Wolfe
   cheiloplasty, W.
   graft, W.
   ptosis operation, W.
Wolff technique
Wolfram syndrome
Wolfring glands
wood tongue blade
Wood procedure
wooden tongue
Woodruff nasopalatine plexus
Woods tonsillar scissors
Woodside procedure
Woodward antral raspatory
woody thyroiditis
Wookey
   neck flap, W.
   pharyngoesophageal reconstruction, w.
   skin tube, w.
Woolner tip
word
   deafness, w.
   debris, w.

word *(continued)*
   salad, w.
   working contact
Wort antral retractor
W-plasty
Wreden sign
Wright
   nasal snare, W.
   quilting stitch, W.
   respirometer, W.
wrinkle
wrinkled
   skin, w.
   tongue, w.
wrinkling
Wrisberg
   cartilage, W.
   nerve, W.
wryneck
W-22 test
Wullstein
   bur, W.
   ear forceps, W.
   ear self-retaining retractor, W.
   handpiece, W.
   knife, W.
   procedure, W.
   retractor, W.
   transplant spatula, W.
   tympanoplasty, W.
Wullstein-House forceps
Wullstein-Zollner tympanoplasty
Wurzburg titanium
   mandibular reconstruction system, W.
   mini bone plate system, W.
   orthognathic implant system, W.
W-V palatal repositioning
W-Y retroposition technique
Wynn
   cleft lip operation, W.
Wynne-Evans tonsil dissector

XYZ

xanthelasma
xanthelasmoidea
xanthodont
xanthodontia
xanthosis
    septum nasi, x. of
X-bite
xenogeneic graft
xenograft
xenophonia
xenorexia
xenotransplantation
Xerac gel
xerocheilia
xeromycteria
xerosialography
xerosis
xerostomia
xerotic
Xomed
    Audiant bone conductor, X.
    Doyle nasal airway splint, X.
    endotracheal tube, X.
    prosthesis, X.
Xomed-Doyle nasal airway splint
x-ray
    bite-wing x.
x-ray goiter
Xylocaine
Y angle
Yaeger lid plate
YAG laser
Yankauer
    antral punch, Y.
    bronchoscope, Y.
    catheter, Y.
    ear curette, Y.
    esophagoscope, Y.
    ethmoid-cutting forceps, Y.
    eustachian instruments, Y.
    laryngoscope, Y.
    middle meatus cannula, Y.
    nasopharyngeal speculum, Y.

Yankauer *(continued)*
    nasopharyngoscope, Y.
    operation, Y.
    pharyngeal speculum, Y.
    probe, Y.
    punch, Y.
    speculum, Y.
    suction tube, Y.
    tonsillar scissors, Y.
    washing tube, Y.
yawn
yawning
Y-axis
Y-closure
yellow
    spot, y.
    teeth, y.
Y-incision
yoke
    mandible, y. of
    maxilla, y. of
Y organ
Yoshida tonsil dissector
Young
    otoplasty, Y.
    tongue-seizing forceps, Y.
Y-suture
Yudin esophagoplasty
Zang space
Zaufal sign
Z'd
Zeis glands
zeisian
Zeiss operating microscope
Zenker
    diverticulum, Z.
    pharyngoesophageal diverticulum, Z.
zero-degree teeth
Z-flap
Ziegler lacrimal probe
zigzag bilateral cleft lip repair
zigzagplasty
Zimany flap

Zimberg esophageal hiatal retractor
zinc
    oxide eugenol, z. (ZOE)
    oxide eugenol cement, z.
    phosphate, z.
    phosphate cement, z.
Z-line of esophagus
ZOE (zinc oxide eugenol)
    dental sealant, Z.
Zoellner
    hook, z.
    raspatory, Z.
    stapes hook, Z.
zones of Schreger
zoograft
zosteroid
Zovickian nape-of-the-neck flap
Z-plastied
Z-plasty
Z-spring
Zuckerkandl gland
Zyclast
Zyderm
zygia (pl. of zygion)
zygion (pl. zygia)
zygoma
    elevator, z.
zygomatic
    arch, z.
    bone, z.
    crest, z.

zygomatic *(continued)*
    process, z.
    reflex, z.
    region, z.
    suture line, z.
zygomaticoauricularis
zygomaticofacial
    canal, z.
    foramen, z.
    nerve, z.
zygomaticofrontal
    suture, z.
zygomaticomaxillary
    fracture, z.
    suture, z.
zygomatico-orbital
    foramen, z.
    suture, z.
zygomaticosphenoid
zygomaticotemporal
    foramen, z.
    suture, z.
zygomaticum
zygomaticus
    muscle, z.
    nerve, z.
zygomaxillare
zygomaxillary
    point, z.
Zylik procedure
ZY-plasty

Additional entries